Rise Above THE CHAOS

How to Keep Positive in
an Unsettled World

CAROLYN GROSS

NEW YORK

LONDON • NASHVILLE • MELBOURNE • VANCOUVER

Rise Above the Chaos

How to Keep Positive in an Unsettled World

Published in New York, New York, by Morgan James Publishing. Morgan James is a trademark of Morgan James, LLC. www.MorganJamesPublishing.com

ISBN 9781642793864 paperback
ISBN 9781642793871 eBook
Library of Congress Control Number: 2018914162

Cover and Interior Design by:
Christopher Kirk
www.GFSstudio.com

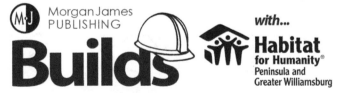

Morgan James is a proud partner of Habitat for Humanity Peninsula and Greater Williamsburg. Partners in building since 2006.

Get involved today! Visit
MorganJamesPublishing.com/giving-back

Disclaimer

Carolyn Gross, the author, is not a healthcare provider or physician. The information in this book should not be construed as "medical advice." The author is merely presenting her findings as would an investigative journalist. Thus, the material in this book should be used for educational and informational purposes only. Each person must make his or her own decisions.

This book details the author's personal experiences with and opinions about addressing unexpected life events that create major life changes, chaos, and stress. The author and publisher are providing this book and its contents on an "as is" basis and make no representations or warranties of any kind with respect to this book or its contents. The author and publisher disclaim all such representations and warranties, including for example warranties of merchantability and healthcare for a particular purpose. In addition, the author and publisher do not represent or warrant that the information accessible via this book is accurate, complete, or current.

The statements made about products and services have not been evaluated by the U.S. Food and Drug Administration. They are not intended to diagnose, treat, cure, or prevent any condition or disease. Please consult with your own physician or healthcare specialist regarding the suggestions and recommendations made in this book.

Except as specifically stated in this book, neither the author nor publisher, nor any authors, contributors, or other representatives will be liable for damages arising out of or in connection with the use of this book. This is a comprehensive limitation of liability that applies to all damages of any kind, including (without limitation) compensatory; direct, indirect, or consequential damages; loss of data, income, or profit; loss of or damage to property; and claims of third parties.

Some names and identifying details have been changed to protect the privacy of individuals. A conscientious effort has been made to only present information that is accurate and truthful in this book. However, the author cannot be held responsible for inaccuracies that may be found in her source material.

This book is not intended as a substitute for consultation with a licensed healthcare practitioner, such as your physician or therapist. Before you begin any health improvement or healthcare regiment that involves changes to your lifestyle in any way, you should consult your physician or another licensed healthcare practitioner to ensure that you are in good health.

Rise Above the Chaos

Table of Contents

Acknowledgements

My highest praise and appreciation goes to my husband, Bryan, who has consistently been patient and offered a support so rare to find in this world. Thank you for coming into my life at the perfect time and for growing with me. You are my partner for Rising Above the Chaos. Having your love and God's love are the things that lift me up.

My heartfelt thanks to my father, Carl F. Sielaff Jr., and my grandfather, Carl F. Sielaff Sr., for always believing in me and treating me like I was gifted and intelligent. I love you both for being entrepreneurs, teachers, and hard workers who wanted to *pass it on*! Also, Christine P. Olfs, the best grandmother a girl could ask for: fashionable, nurturing, and blonde into her nineties.

I want to thank my California Sister Terry Jelley for unwavering friendship as we explore our spiritual purposes. Also, for the best place to write in Southern California. I treasure our holidays together and having a safe haven to restore, relax and renew myself while writing.

Working with Geronimo Rubio, MD, has been an amazing journey as well. His ability to stay levelheaded and heal cases that others wouldn't even take on has been miraculous to witness. His Immunotherapy protocols saved my life fifteen years ago when I was diagnosed with breast cancer, thank you compadre.

Just love and adore my work team that keeps me on track; Tram Nguyen, Jamie Ravard, and Bao Phan. Plus, the kindness and insights of my personal trainer, Mark Arjona.

Heartfelt appreciation to the team at Morgan James Publishing: David, Jim, Terry, Aubrey, Bonnie and the designers and sales associates. You all make a difference!

My life has been accented by influences from many ministers, healers, and friends who helped me reconstruct my soul and life. I adore and respect you: Rev. Judith Larkin Reno PhD, Ken Sutherland, Ann Meyer Makeever, Roberta Zito, Sandra Orchin, Sandra Lee, Jennifer Allen Prather, and lots of Reverends: Kayla Rose Carroll, Elizabeth Brabant, Mary Ann Kelley, Brigette Heimers, Brian and Sheila Anderson to name a few!

Grateful to the many health professionals and advocates who inspire me to continue to fight for health solutions and patient rights: Frank Cousineau, Ann Fonfa, Ellen Jensen, Annie Brandt, and Barbara Evans.

Thank you for the Grace of God; keeping me and my dreams alive, to bring this message into the world!

Introduction

This book is designed for unexpected life events. Those events that come out of left field and make you question everything you thought you knew about yourself and the world around you. It's the phone call from the doctor or the hit-and-run accident. It's the chaos of losing a child or bearing witness to horrific images in the news that bring you right back to unresolved traumas in your life.

The tools and stories shared in this book are here to help you navigate through life's turbulent waters as well as lift your spirits and enliven your soul. Rising above the chaos in the midst of life's most challenging moments calls for a game plan, and that's just what this book is. It's designed to be read right in the midst of the most chaotic storms or in the light at first dawn when you have the time to process the messages the Universe is sending your way.

This I know for sure: game-changer chaos doesn't send a text, postcard, or IM. It just shows up! How prepared you are to react depends on a number of variables, but *self-knowledge,* managing your internal chaos, and *self-care* are the building blocks you will need for a successful landing, and they are a few of the main concepts in this book.

There are different kinds of chaos: internal and external. When it involves health, money, and family or cherished relationships, it's often internal chaos that hits home. When the disruption is Mother Nature demolishing your house or losing your job, it's external chaos, and it's time for a new beginning. Actually, almost every chaotic, game-changer, unexpected event gives you a new beginning: either immediately or somewhere down the road.

This book is meant to be a friend and guide to help you navigate through the wreckage so you can find your new beginning. The most important first step in any traumatic blow is to bolster your self-care and self-confidence. When everything seems against you and chaos is winning, it's time for a motivational speech. A personal pep talk to convince yourself, early in the crisis, that you are ready for this. If the diagnosis, job change, or relationship loss is too much to look at, don't look at the problem until you are ready. Your first step is to remind yourself of your resiliency, before any problem solving can occur.

Look to this book as a roadmap to help show you the way to navigate in uncertain times, through stories, tools, and thoughtful insights into how important you are. I mean the "real you" and not your social media mask. Chaos makes us confront what we want in life and what's truly important. This book will reintroduce *you* to *you* so that you know how much your life matters. Again, I mean your real life with your family and friends.

Chaos makes these questions rise to the surface. As you search for your personal truth, be aware of what social media and the internet are trying to sell you. Truth gets a bad rap lately, as if there is no absolute truth. Fight against that trend. We have to learn to decipher the truth. You can still detect it in the way you feel when you read about something or someone. Truth is still relevant and meaningful. Seek it out.

If you are new to inner reflection, there's nothing better in the world to set you on that fulfilling path than game-changing chaos. It is our biggest teacher and tests us by fire. And the prize for surviving these tests is self-knowledge. Once we're out of the cauldron, we know our strengths and weaknesses.

It was my intention, when I set out to write and publish a similar book in 2002, to help people who are going through unexpected ordeals, where they felt unequipped for the problem at hand. I thought I had already learned plenty of those tough lessons when I wrote *Staying Calm in the Midst of Chaos*, the earlier version of this book, but I was wrong. The original manuscript was crafted from my work as a craniosacral therapist (a form of alternative therapy using gentle touch) and my religious and esoteric studies. It was written before the events of September 11, 2001. However, as the country dealt with its collective grief and anger, it became apparent that my book had an audience and a purpose.

In 2002, I published *Staying Calm in the Midst of Chaos* and went on an eighteen-month, twenty-four-city book tour. It was in Cleveland, Ohio that game-changer chaos showed up again in my life, this time disguised as a large lump in my left breast. The book tour was put on the shelf when I was diagnosed with Stage 3 Infiltrating Ductal Carcinoma. I had to pivot my energies to the chaos in my own internal world, healing stage 3 breast cancer.

The treatment was successful, and I used several strategies from the first edition of my *Staying Calm* book. One of my favorites was "The Better I Know Myself, the Better I Show Myself," because I knew I was exhausted from the book tour and travel before my diagnosis. When they wanted to do a mastectomy, chemo, and radiation in FULL DOSES … I ran scared. That meant I had to find another way to heal—which I did.

In 2003, I used immunotherapy and LOW DOSES of chemo and radiation. This book is not my cancer story, as I've written two books on that topic: *Treatable and Beatable: Healing Cancer without Surgery* and *Breaking the Cancer Code: A Revolutionary Approach to Reversing Cancer*, co-authored by Geronimo Rubio, MD.

After I healed from cancer using my own immune system and targeted T-cell treatments called vaccines, the next lesson arrived from chaos, the great teacher. I had the opportunity to help other cancer patients professionally, and I did so for over a decade as they "tried out" this new, non-invasive therapy. My work as a patient advocate was gratifying and meaningful, but it also acted like a grindstone on me. I worked with individuals and their families with mostly stage 4 cancer. These high-stakes situations were with people who needed constant attention and made enormous demands, and it stretched me further in keeping my own internal chaos at bay.

Now a cancer survivor with new insights into chaos and abuse, I poured myself into crafting an updated and revised version of my earlier work. This time I had over twenty-five years of research working with all kinds of patients and coaching clients in the midst of chaos. Their stories, as well as my experiences, are woven into this book. I heard that it takes 10,000 hours to be successful in a craft, and I've put that and more into this book for you.

When you get kerfuffled, this book will ground you in your truth by questioning who you are in the world and your place within it. I want to help you be ready and understand that whatever you are experiencing isn't a personal vendetta the Universe has plotted against you. No, it's just another lesson to grow you stronger.

I'll suggest the concept of being a "grow-getter," using your obstacle to help you grow greater and stay afloat in whatever lesson you are in right now. Whatever you are facing today, know that you can turn that hurt, confusion, anger, distrust, upset, and angst into something positive and life-affirming. I promise I've got you.

The first half of the book will define chaos and outline the emotional and mental health issues surrounding it, with lots of personal and client stories to illuminate key concepts.

Then, the second half of the book will offer concrete tools and techniques to transform chaos from something negative to something positive. I offer these stories and exercises as a bright light to travel with so you will know that you can take concrete steps to neutralize chaos—to be more proactive and less reactive to what life throws at us all. You will learn what you can and cannot control and how to resolve to undo any internal chaos getting in your way.

No matter what is facing you today, I hope you find purpose and a sense of strength in whatever you chose to do. Let's take that first step to heal together.

Chapter 1
Chaos: The Great Teacher

There is more to life than increasing its speed.
~Gandhi

N
o matter how confident some people may appear, no one breezes through life. The *great teacher* can start in our early years or, for others, it's waiting in the future. No matter when or where chaos intersects with our lives, there are times when we all become overwhelmed, make mistakes, and fall. Overextended, under-staffed, overtired, or under-appreciated: these words all conjure up images of chaos. Unexpected circumstances don't send an email or text message; they just show up!

Chaos is an equal opportunity offender. Whatever your position in life, turmoil knows no bounds and offers no guarantees. Whether you are highly successful or struggling with the basics, everyone has to pay the price when internal or external chaos leads them astray. Add to that today's transparent world with so much disclosure: even those who thought their deeds had stayed under wraps below the radar can no longer assume such privilege.

In our advanced society with technology connecting us continually to greater frontiers, we find ourselves facing historic levels of stress from real or imagined situations, events, and threats, from the now all-too-common school shooting to random acts of terrorism both large and small. Learning not just to survive but also thrive in our turbulent times means learning how to manage both internal and external chaos. The good news: you can learn how to harness havoc for personal growth. Let's first look at the different types of scenarios.

External Chaos

External chaos lives front and center in our lives. It's a call to action that can't be ignored, whether it's a doctor's diagnosis or a hurricane on the horizon. We experience it in our jobs and in the extensive roles we play in our personal lives. External chaos shows in our health dynamics and in the way we connect with others professionally and privately. External turmoil can bring us to our knees and test the resiliency of any relationships.

Add to this the external influences of media mania. Without noticing, we are often fed bad news from breakfast to bedtime. In the news business, the mantra "if it bleeds, it leads" is what matters most. So, it's no surprise that our social media feeds, with both local and national news, are focused on the most negative and salacious aspects of life; our timelines are full of reports of school bullying, workplace harassment, domestic violence, and racism. The media focuses on our differences and not on what unites us. Because the media is exposing and manipulating the worst of our tribal natures, we find ourselves feeling out of control and stressed. No one wants to be diagnosed with cancer, find out his or her relationship is over online, or be scammed out of retirement. The backdrop of living has changed dramatically in recent decades because of how we are digitally connected.

A click away can be bad news about a loved one or friend. These external scenarios create distraction and concerns. Then there's the impact of social media that amplifies what we are already reacting to daily as we absorb news in political and public situations, catastrophic events by Mother Nature, or terrorists. All these external events concern us and can trigger the most unsuspecting person.

Instead of saving us precious time, this high-tech world adds labor to our lives. We may no longer lick stamps and address envelopes, but now we must respond to e-mails and answer text messages and cell phones around the clock, as we try to keep up with the information overload. We sometimes get results by flipping a switch, but we must also contend with our computers being hacked, cell phones that get lost, and equipment that diabolically goes on the blink at the worst possible time. These situations are commonplace, and we rarely learn how to handle the resulting stress until we're desperate.

Internal Chaos

Internal chaos is not a middle-of-the-road situation. It lives on the fringes but permeates every aspect of our lives. External events can trigger internal loss or abandonment. Based on what we've lived through, we have a backdrop that acts as a filter to all our life events. For many of us, it's a personal or health-related crisis that finally forces us to look at our internal chaos issues. Heart attack survivors are classic examples of those who make lifestyle changes under duress. Many experts speculate that over ninety percent of all illnesses are stress related. No wonder: the miracles of technology have forced us to become multi-taskers and multi-role players.

Figuring out how to discern the truth and communicate with people is becoming another complex scenario that we internalize. If "fake news" has made it online and on the airways, what is the payoff for truth-telling? Inner turmoil is minimal when we tell the truth, think kind thoughts, and extend random acts of kindness. Internal chaos is quelled from giving, not taking, and from allowing things to unfold rather than exerting hypervigilant control. These attributes—kindness, truth-telling, and relinquishing control—are not typically celebrated in our society. However, if you aim to lessen internal chaos, these skills are literal lifesavers.

It's like the world is set on crisis mode these days and if we overreact, then we are making our own internal environment worse. Most of the strategies in this book are going to help you with managing your internal chaos so you can bring calm into your situation and be the change you want to see in the world. It all starts with self-management. Addressing your internal chaos is a monumental task today because life is complicated, but self-awareness is simple. Good self-care and awareness skills can create balance or homeostasis to help you rise above the chaos.

Pain: When Is It a Warning?

Even those who think they aren't achieve-aholics often take dreams of peace to their graves—or to the hospital—because they never made time for serenity during their vital years. One of my clients, a high-profile beauty salon owner, was working twelve-hour days in her shop while saddled with administrative duties. She came to me complaining of neck pain so intense that she couldn't turn her head.

"My neck hurts all the time," she explained. "I work on people's heads all day, and now my head is killing me. Can you do anything?"

Having worked as an executive coach, patient advocate, and craniosacral therapist, I was thrilled to be able to answer yes. The effects of constant chaos are very physical. According to the American Medical Association, it's well-known that during times of stress, the sympathetic nervous system prevails. That means the heart rate rises, vessels widen to increase blood flow, glucose levels are elevated, saliva and gastric acid production diminishes, gastrointestinal activity ceases, and skeletal muscle strength intensifies. Translated, this means the heart races, digestion stops, adrenaline secretion is high, and the body is ready for action.

During rest, the parasympathetic system dominates as we rebuild and release. The heart rate decreases, digestive processes are stimulated, and gastrointestinal elimination is activated. This is where homeostasis and life balance happen. Allowing ourselves to rest is restorative and necessary to heal from tumultuous times.

As a result of nerve activity, tensions caused by internal and external chaos are frequently stored in the core of the body: the head, neck, and spine. In the practice of yoga, massage, acupuncture, or craniosacral therapy, those are the areas we focus on and address since they activate the parasympathetic nervous system. The gentle manipulations during treatment or stretching allow stored tensions to unwind. As this pressure is released, the body begins to heal and balance itself.

When working with clients, I found a striking correlation between mind and body functions. Shoulder and neck pain, for example, often occurs when people take on too much *responsibility*. Dental problems surface from clenched jaws or stress-eating, while back ailments tend to strike those who lack support or feel financially insecure. For my hairdresser client, her pace of life was literally a pain in the neck. She was so focused on being a successful business owner that she ignored her body's cry for help. During her consultation, I urged her to slow down.

"You clearly need more time off," I counseled. "I can get your neck in great shape in a few sessions, but if you don't make some changes, you'll be wasting your money."

Pain is a great motivator for us all. If you are facing continual frustrations and challenges, don't blame everyone else; see what it is you need to do or change. My salon owner desperately wanted to feel better. She began by cutting back her hours and hiring an additional stylist. The salon still netted the same money, and she now felt happier and healthier. I can't tell you how many people I've worked with who found that when they reduced their work/life stress and increased their exercise, relaxation, bodywork, and leisure time, they still managed to maintain their income while improving their lifestyle. Trust me; it can be done!

When we allow time for the parasympathetic system to restore us, we have more clarity. With all the activities clamoring for attention, clarity is often not valued. We place more emphasis on continual productivity than healthy boundaries and self-care. Yet, according to Brian Tracy, one of the most celebrated lifestyle authors and educators of today, eighty percent of goal achievement is due to clarity.

What is the Price of Success?

When the vast majority of people experience a near-fatal illness or accident, they rarely regret the unreturned business phone call or an uncompleted sales report. Instead, they lament time not spent with loved ones, canceled vacations, and unfulfilled passions.

This principle calls to mind a successful real estate mogul hell-bent on making his first million by 30 years old. Pushing himself to the limit, he managed to fulfill his boyhood dream. After three decades, he had it all: money, power, a lovely wife, and four children. Then, he collapsed. His breakdown was so severe that he was unable to return to work for two years. Bedridden with depression, he had plenty of time to reflect on the high cost of his rich-and-famous fantasies. In time, he was able to parlay his story into a book, and he began speaking to audiences on "How to Succeed without Burnout." Ben Kubassek eventually returned to work, and today his life is prospering. He's happy and fulfilled, *and* he has learned the invaluable lesson of working without pushing over the precipice into chaos.

Why is managing chaos and stress such a hot topic today? It's because most of us need permission to slow down and pay attention to our needs. Many of us push ourselves into sixty-hour work weeks while raising our families, taking classes, keeping fit, trying to look young, and winning the occasional award. We go, go, go … but do we know where we are going? Someone once said, "If life is a race, then the finish line is the graveyard."

My goal in writing this book was to convince people to make lifestyle adjustments and self-care choices, so they enjoy not just success, but their lives. One of the chief indicators of chaos is a body that feels out of alignment. When we go into crisis mode, the body's homeostasis is thrown off balance. This may manifest itself in the form of neck pain, headaches, digestive problems, chronic back or shoulder aches, fatigue, or depression. Also, a body chronically out of balance will eventually succumb to heart disease, cancer, high blood pressure, obesity, and digestive problems.

We cannot control one hundred percent of the events in our lives, but we can control the way we respond. The key is learning to recognize the difference so that we spend our limited emotional resources on what we can control and let the other stuff go. We cannot guarantee that our loved ones—or we ourselves—will always be healthy, nor can we predict our financial future or job success. One health crisis or lawsuit can blow a retirement account. However, no matter what curve balls knock us for a loop, we *can* master our response to these events. To me, the only safety net we truly have is how we act and react to what life serves up.

This is how chaos becomes the great teacher—we learn in the midst of a crisis just how strong we really are. Sometimes, we find more inner resources than we give ourselves credit for; other times, we discover our vulnerabilities. Often, when we embark on a new enterprise—a new home or business, a relationship, a creative project—we find surprising reserves of energy and enthusiasm that enable us to achieve that first heady feeling of success.

Then one day we wake up and feel less passion and drive. We may notice that we're relying on unhealthy lifestyle choices to sustain us—too many lattes and high-calorie snacks by day and more than a social drink to unwind at night. We can get away with these habits for a while, but eventually these crutches will age us before our time. Chaos always catches up to us. The minute we realize that we're using quick fixes to get through our daily routine (Starbucks anyone?), it's time to reevaluate our life's choices.

I once heard about an actress who simultaneously starred in a hit TV series by day and had the leading role in a Broadway play at night. It seemed a nearly superhuman feat. *What a woman!* However, on a television talk show, she confessed that she had become a caffeine junkie, downing seven or eight cups of coffee a day. I couldn't help thinking, *what a role model for unhealthy living.* I haven't heard much about her lately, but I do hope she's managed to survive. Excessive caffeine and chaos go together. Neither allows the parasympathetic activity the time it needs to rebuild and rest.

When I work one-on-one with clients or speak at conferences, I introduce several strategies to equip those seeking balance to offset the impact of internal versus external chaos. I guide individuals through an exercise where they review a list of stress symptoms. If someone has two or three symptoms, I inform them that they're in the right room and need to pay attention to the program. It is not uncommon for people to report as many as ten or more symptoms of stress out of a possible twenty. This is a clear indicator of a health problem waiting to happen. (See the Symptom of Stress Quiz in Chapter 3.)

Unfortunately, many of us have been learning from the *great teacher* since childhood. Adverse childhood experiences (emotional, physical, or sexual abuse) strengthen those who survive them. It's the positive side of such a negative experience. Being forged by early childhood trauma steels us in strength and resiliency if we're willing to look inward. However, even if you had the most terrific childhood, unexpected circumstances later in life that seem unsettling can leave a lasting damaging imprint on our lives.

How do we turn tragedy into triumph or rejection into perfection? We start by redefining our life lessons and trusting the process through whatever chaos is yet unresolved, knowing it will correct itself one day. This takes trust and patience, but I promise you it's worth every effort.

Once armed with the various techniques offered in this book, you can engage in the challenges of our fast-paced, achieve-success society and contribute to the world without sacrificing your happiness, health, and legacy. The path is available when you permit yourself to value your health and your heart enough to make lifestyle adjustments before stress evolves into serious, chronic illness. This change requires an important shift to looking at the lessons being taught by the turmoil in your life. That's the purpose of this book: to offer you support to help you rise above the chaos, stay calm, and prioritize your life. Now, let's dive into the different categories of chaos.

Chapter 2
Categories of Chaos

Your adversity is your advantage. It builds muscles, not wounds.
~Darren Hardy

Chaos comes in many forms, and the first step in rising above chaos is learning to identify and recognize its many faces. That's what this chapter is all about. It's precisely in moments of personal or professional upheaval where we need to define and confront the nature of the evil beast. When our abstract analytical mind grabs hold of a fearful situation, we can be overwhelmed by problems in all areas. Real or imagined, these thoughts activate all our stress hormones. If these fear storms take over, we are completely out of the moment.

Think back on a situation where you were waiting for a loved one to arrive, and when he or she failed to show up, you began thinking the worst. Suddenly, your whole being became upset, restless, and fitful, and the tension lasted until your fears were proved unfounded. Sound familiar? That's the insidious nature of internal chaos. One thought leads to another until we're overwhelmed and convinced the worst has happened, even if we have no actual data to prove it.

I like to give people a point of reference if they have lots of obsessive thoughts swirling, to help ground them to reality. Below is a list of categories of chaos you can use like a barometer. If you're feeling stressed and your internal chaos temperature is running high, or you feel a "storm" pending, you can reference why, and course correct. When I'm overreacting to some situation, I will run through this checklist to assess where I need to make some adjustments to regain my composure. The better I know myself, the better I show myself.

1) Too Many Commitments Causes Confusion

We are go-getters here in America, which is great until we lose our brilliant decision-making capacity or practical perspective. One of my former bosses was a motivated and ambitious executive who always had ten or more projects going simultaneously. If he was functioning well, no problem; his sales team could follow his directives. However, as soon as he got overwhelmed with worry or jittery from all his responsibilities, his staff would derail as well. But if he was out of sorts, he'd project his frustrations and micromanage his seasoned professionals (see Category Two: Resentments for how that worked out. Hint: not well!).

One day I advised him, "You're like the spoke in a wheel, and everything revolves around you. So, when you lose focus and get anxious about projects, we do too." Overachievers need to be warned not to *be* the category of chaos to their staff or families—especially for people who thrive on productivity.

2) Resentments: Prisons Without Walls

We can all ruminate on the hurts and slights we receive in life. Our brains can get stuck looking in the rearview mirror, focused on past resentments instead of plans and positivity. When we're obsessed with recent stings and perceived injustices, we can get mired in the muck instead of rising above it. Simply stated, hate hurts the hater. Those who have caused and created the injustice aren't suffering when you send them negative thoughts; resentments bounce back every time, contaminating your mental airspace.

One of my favorite examples of all time happened when I spoke at a women's conference in Antelope Valley, California. A nun named Sister Antonia came to pray for the speakers at a special dinner the night before the event. This isn't commonplace in a non-sectarian event, but it happened.

As this sixty-something nun calmly and methodically made her way to the podium, I felt drawn to her. I noticed her shoulders slightly hunched forward like she had been praying most of her life. Before she launched into her prayer, she shared something about herself.

She spoke about her ministry to serve inmates and that this role led her to live with the inmates at the prison herself. Well, that got everyone's attention. She then told us that her mission was to help those inmates with life sentences to heal themselves of their resentments.

Let's face it: they probably had deeper resentments than you and me, right? Her next statement was nearly as shocking. Sister Antonia told us that she is always surprised when she does public work outside the prison and finds people in the free world who are unhappier than her incarcerated clients.

She said, "So many people that are free, living their lives without bars, are confined by their resentments and are living in prisons without walls."

I had never heard of a better definition of resentments in my life! And I'd been seeking something memorable for years. Resentments are like me putting myself behind bars. So, let me ask you: Do you want to live confined by your resentments? If not, it's in your power to find a key and let yourself out of your self-imposed cell. To forgive is divine, but it doesn't mean you will ever forget.

3) Illness Reveals Inexperience

The most unsuspecting people can be walking around thinking life is easy-breezy and then, suddenly, a diagnosis changes everything. In my role as a survivor and patient advocate for the last fifteen years, I have seen firsthand how disruptive a diagnosis can be, especially for someone who has never paid attention to his or her health before.

I remember a woman who worked in my office who was cute, smart, ambitious, and finding her way in the world in her mid-thirties. She had it all going on, including a handsome husband, to boot.

Then they had their first child, and he was diagnosed with autism. This mother poured all her smarts and determination into helping her child.

Refusing to accept what the doctors had outlined for her child's future, she started on a holistic approach to address symptoms, including putting her son on a strict, healthy diet. The next thing you know, all her talent and time was focused exclusively on improving her child's life. It was chaos for her as she lost sleep and serenity; she began fraying at the ends. However, she was grateful for the eye-opening experience because her life used to be focused on external success, and now she knew more about what truly mattered in life. She connected more with mothers facing these same challenges then she ever had with her work family.

4) Procrastination

We all have deadlines, both personal and professional. Deadlines put pressure on us to perform, whether it's planning a wedding, submitting a college application, applying for a grant, or just plain old tax time. Deadlines have this impending imprint we sometimes put off because it's not due today. However, today comes, and we're often ill-prepared and have to move mountains to make our commitments. Procrastination causes chaos. If you have a big presentation or paper to write, thinking about it causes stress, whereas being proactive diminishes it. In the moment, we believe procrastination is helping us, only to find out later that it's working against us. Delay causes us more worry than if we'd just put on our grownup pants and done the work before it was due.

Procrastinating about decisions causes chaos too—especially the big decisions. *Should I stay at this job or school? What about this man or woman, are they right for my future or ruining it? What about staying single, do I still try to find a partner? Should I start my own business or get into a partnership?* The list is endless, and depending on where you are in your life, you can be procrastinating about what to do with parents, children, or other family members who need some support. Chaos multiplies as we delay.

5) Loss of the Familiar

Life is about change. Even when people stay with the same partner or company for extended periods of time, change happens. Mergers and acquisitions can take us by surprise, and when they are announced, employees often wonder, "Why all the new rules?" As soon as the merger is official, they get why. Hopefully, work is only a portion of your life, but no one escapes tough times. We all must navigate the loss of relationships, family, friends, and neighbors. Each loss impacts us with concerns as we wonder: what will happen next? So, when the familiar sands of your life are shifting, you have to have self-assurance. While writing this book, I got my own game-changing surprise. I was working with a client on an annual contract, and the organization wanted to change the terms dramatically, none of which were beneficial or respectful to me. Immediately, I realized this was hitting on all of the big three chaos areas at once: health, money, and relationships. My first step was self-care: it was just too early to look at all the possible fallout. No way; it was too disorienting. I needed to take a long walk on the beach. And there, in the sunset, I spent several hours remembering how all my big-chaos game-changers had pushed me forward. Leaving home in my youth. Cancer. Career missteps. Each and every one had, once the dust settled, moved me to bigger and better opportunities. So, if your life is messy and chaotic, hold on for the ride and use the experience to fall forward.

Be a *grow* getter. Stop looking out the windshield or into the future all the time; instead, take a look into the rearview mirror. What past losses have you had that seemed, at the moment, like impending threats, only to find everything worked out and settled just fine? Bring that confidence into this moment. Sometimes it's best to make a journal of all the shifting situations and losses you've been through. Make a list and then ask: What gift did each give you? Perhaps a new job or a healthier approach to life. Aging is a loss of the familiar too, because we may feel great inside, but our bodies don't take the abuse of youth.

Many who read this have no concern of that loss, but if you're lucky enough to grow old, someday you will. One of the gifts of my mother was that she was a fabulous example of aging gracefully, and she wisely stated, "Each decade, we learn something new!"

So, if you're entering a new decade with concern, turn it around.

6) Criticism and Condemnation

Having someone judge you and see you as inept, difficult, or not as "good" as they are causes lots of problems too. The highest principled people do not embody this. I can't help but think of the Dalai Lama, someone so kind and ready to end human suffering through peace, compassion, and love. With all his worldly status, he doesn't act as if he's better than us. He models the exact opposite.

It may surprise you that those who are judging us create as much chaos for themselves as those who are being criticized and condemned. It's hard to remember this, especially at the moment. If we feel a lack of support or are called out for no reason, this, of course, causes inner doubt and confusion. Confronted with criticism and condemnation, we wonder: *why am I being isolated or treated as a second-rate citizen?* I know this hurts in the moment.

However, if we take a step back, we can see that our critic is also filled with negativity. When someone acts superior and implies you are not welcome or worthy by their conversation or body language, they shut off their kindness; their goodness is turned off when they shun you. Remember that with resentments, hate hurts the hater; and that hurt people hurt others.

7) Worry and Fear

One key to lessening worry and fear is remembering that the future is in bigger hands than yours. Also, the more you worry about life's factors that you can't control, the more havoc and uncertainty you'll face. Chaos and fear are closely linked. Shifting into a panic state fuels the flames of chaos. I love the term "fear storms," because that is what they are, and, eventually, the fear will blow over just like a storm, if we don't encourage it to stay. As life moves us along, we sometimes find ourselves vulnerable when we don't understand new and unfamiliar situations, from the latest technology to new parenting approaches or co-working situations. The future is unknown and uncertain, and this is another culprit of tumult. However, when you "awfulize" what is potentially ahead, you ruin the present. When you move to a new city, get a new job, negotiate a promotion, have a baby, or find out someone is unkindly gossiping about you … how do you find your center? By focusing on the factors in your favor or in your control.

The stress of living in worry or fear releases lots of chemicals into our bodies that aren't productive in the long-term. Your fight-or-flight response may save you in a car accident but activating those levels of adrenaline every day of your commute is problematic. As a country, so many of our citizens are exposed to traumatic events, whether it's as a veteran of combat or a survivor of incest. These walking survivors often have PTSD, which highlights our human need to repair after extensive exposure to duress.

How do you repair? Some people use faith and prayer, which we will delve into more in the chapters that follow. Others use positive expectations and affirmations, and it's also helpful to use physical activity to stop the runaway-train brain. Taking walks with friends and letting your concerns go, even for a brief respite, can work wonders. Texting friends or journaling is a release for many, too. However you communicate, the purpose is to vent your concerns, and if the fear and worry don't quiet down, see a counselor or minister, or work with a coach.

As you work through the rest of the book, please keep these seven categories of chaos in the front of your mind. These are the factors that create internal or external stress that has to be managed or else it shows up as illness, mental suffering, and strained relationships. In the next chapter, we'll look at how to identify how your body is holding up to the external environment and processing the impact chaos has on you.

Chapter 3
Symptoms of Stress

The greatest weapon against stress is our ability
to choose one thought over another.
~William James

We need to acquaint ourselves with the symptoms of stress for one fundamental reason: *prevention.* Corporations now realize how important it is to reboot the batteries of their teams, so annual meetings frequently have a workplace-wellness component. Even the hotels where these events are taking place offer the use of the spa and yoga or mindfulness classes to give an added benefit to their clientele. Managers should understand that if they don't mentor their staff by example in taking care of themselves, their bottom line suffers.

When we pay attention to stress symptoms and stop popping antidepressants and stimulants, we can prevent illness and imbalance, as well as increase job performance. I once had a boss who would take non-drowsy cold medication just for the energy boost. Can you relate? What is *your* quick fix when you feel depleted?

In his book *Spirituality, Stress, and You,* Baptist minister Thomas Rodgerson wrote that he once delivered a sermon at his new parish after staying up half the night to prepare. As the congregation greeted him after the service, a ninety-seven-year-old woman approached him, shook his hand, and said, "You're operating without any reserve of energy. Go home and take a nap before you wear your body out!" Being the astute lady that she was, she ministered to the minister that day.

How often do we ignore our bodies' messages in the form of headaches, fatigue, or flu because we—like that minister—think we must press on? Certainly, there are times when we have no choice, times when situations dictate extraordinary measures. However, there is always a cost. Throughout my career, I've attracted the clients whose pace is to speed through life like racehorses. You know the types—the overachievers who lose sight of their health because the heady winds of success have blown warning signs off the map. My main message is simple: Don't ignore warning signs. You may think you're indestructible, but you are not. I've seen many international executives at the apex of their careers suddenly bedridden by cancer. Certain health challenges level the playing field. We're all susceptible to the symptoms of stress.

Another example is an executive who was interviewed on *60 Minutes*. He was doing damage control for his company because of an automobile recall, and he hadn't had a day off for ten weeks. The footage showed his two young sons, playing at his desk on a Sunday so they could be with their dad. A close-up of the mid-fifty's executive revealed a shingles-like rash all over his face. He looked like a wreck. He was doing what he had to do—but the price was high.

Your Crisis Reserve Account

Like the Minister preparing all night for the sermon or the executive doing damage control for his corporation, the only way we can pull off this kind of feat is to have a reserve account of strength and energy. Whenever we allow the parasympathetic system time to rest and restore us, we are depositing energy to shore us up during times of crisis. Much like money in the bank, you add to this account when you sleep, eat healthy foods, receive massages, or do whatever it is that restores your soul.

For some, it might be hiking, golfing, reading, writing, or even cooking. It doesn't matter what it is; it only matters that you make these life-saving deposits. If you can block out a full day, that's wonderful, but some busy executives and moms on the go can only carve out four- or five-hour blocks of time. Make sure whatever you do fulfills you completely. It's a time to unplug from the responsibilities of your life. My favorite reprieve is the mineral waters in the Palm Springs area. I never leave a visit to the pools without being completely relaxed. There will be additional solutions in Chapter 11 to help you get in check.

When you have a healthy balance in your "crisis reserve account," you're more easily able to handle job or relationship changes, illness, or other calamities. And when a crisis is over, your priority should be to rebuild your reserves, so you'll be ready for the next crisis. Restoration has never been more critical than it is today.

The Impact of Digital Distraction

Technology propels us so fast that we're now expected to communicate almost instantaneously. Most people wake up and immediately check their phone to see who texted, emailed, or called. It's like we aren't awake until we touch our phone and tell the world, *I'm here!* But the need to unplug is suddenly getting new attention and causing renewed interest in the positive power of mindfulness. We have all observed how quiet we've become at airports, restaurants, and public gatherings when we're glued to our phones instead of looking at the people or environment around us. You can observe this on beaches, in restaurants, and at spas. Despite all of the online connection, there is a trend toward loneliness in our world.

At a recent outing with another couple, we were excitedly greeting each other before a day of leisure at the San Diego Zoo when one member of the group decided she had to check in for a flight the next day on her phone. I thought it strange to say hello to the group and then suddenly dive into her digital world while three real-world friends were right in front of her, ready for a day of fun and connection. Clearly, this gal had not unplugged and was oblivious to everyone else in that moment. Patiently we talked around her until she was able to join in without her device in hand.

Information Overload

In another scenario with two other couples attending an event, we were talking and a question came up. Instead of discussing the merits of the question and speculating on the answer, everyone pulled out their phones to do some quick fact-checking though most of us felt like this interrupted the conversation. Do you agree? Is it more enjoyable to have the digital answers instantaneously or be in the moment with conversation and community? Should we spend more time talking to our friends and family versus asking Google or Siri the answers? What are we losing when these digital distractions interrupt our normal conversations? Just because we can access information any time doesn't mean we should. And, if you're looking to control the chaos in your life, your cell phone is a fantastic place to start.

Jeff Davis is a prolific author who speaks about the information base, which used to double every fifteen years. But in the later part of the twentieth century, it increased to every five years, and now in the twenty-first century, according to Buckminster Fuller, the "Knowledge Doubling Curve," he noticed that until 1900 human knowledge doubled approximately every century. By the end of World War II, knowledge was doubling every twenty-five years. Today, things are not as simple since different types of knowledge have different rates of growth. For example, nanotechnology knowledge is doubling every two years and clinical knowledge every eighteeen months. But, on average, human knowledge is doubling every thirteen months. According to IBM, the build-out of the "internet of things" will lead to the doubling of knowledge every twelve hours. Human knowledge doubles nearly every thirteen months, with scientific knowledge following every eighteen months. What happens to our civilization when so much data is constantly flooding our brains? One thing is for sure: We all feel we should be learning more, doing more, posting more, and *being* more. Psychological studies on communicating and resolving conflict are crucial in a society where high school violence and road rage have become daily occurrences.

The good news is that cutting-edge medicine and nutrition have increased our life expectancy, and alternative medicine now offers new options for healing and wellness. But living longer means there's more to learn, so that you can make informed decisions. Financial planning and stock market strategies are now necessary for almost everyone to augment Social Security and savings. And the list goes on and on. It's a question of whether we are driving ourselves or our phones' access is fueling our feelings of anxiety and stress.

So, let's do a little self-evaluation as we look at the symptoms of stress and how they are affecting you. The following quiz will help you identify how you are holding up in the modern world of digital distractions. It will also help determine if, when it comes to aging, you are on the fast track to a big slowdown. Because burnout is near for many of us if we don't reassess our priorities.

Symptoms of Stress Self-Quiz

Answer yes or no to the following questions:

1. I sleep with my phone nearby.

   Yes_____   No_____

2. I get headaches easily.

   Yes_____   No_____

3. I have digestive problems.

   Yes_____   No_____

4. I frequently get colds and flu.

        Yes_____   No_____

5. I often have interrupted sleep or insomnia.

        Yes_____   No_____

6. I always feel rushed.

        Yes_____   No_____

7. I can't remember anything.

        Yes_____   No_____

8. I drive too fast.

        Yes_____   No_____

9. I drink caffeine throughout the day.

        Yes_____   No_____

10. I eat high-fat or sugary foods to boost my energy.

        Yes_____   No_____

11. I'm smoking or vaping more, or I've recently started again.

        Yes_____   No_____

12. I drink more alcohol than I used to.

        Yes_____   No_____

13. I often lose my temper.

        Yes_____   No_____

14. I can't stop thinking about my problems or "shut off" my busy brain.

        Yes_____   No_____

15. I'm carrying a lot of tension in my neck, back, or shoulders.

        Yes_____   No_____

16. I don't have the optimism I once had.

        Yes_____   No_____

17. I often feel fatigued.

        Yes_____   No_____

18. I'm often clumsy; I keep dropping or bumping into things.

Yes_____ No_____

19. I seem to get into more arguments than I used to.

Yes_____ No_____

Now, Count your number of "Yes" responses.

Total Score _____

Score 1-3: I am living wisely and have slowed down the aging process. Living life at this pace is comfortable and rewarding.

Score 4-5: I am in need of some solutions to keep calm. I'm not yet fast-tracking toward old age, but it's time to slow down and see if I can become more effective. I need more quality than quantity in my life.

Score 5-6: My reserves are running low, and solutions to stress need to be a priority. I'm already on the aging fast track but can easily get back in balance by making some lifestyle changes.

Score 7-8: My reserves are almost empty. I need to implement several lifestyle changes, and I need to do it NOW. Continuing as I am will keep me on this fast track to aging.

Score 9-10: I'm running on empty. I need to take time off to rest, to restore my reserves, and to reevaluate my life's priorities so I can implement much-needed change.

Score 11-13: I've been functioning on empty for a while, maybe years. I probably need professional help to restore my health. Acupuncture, massage, and chiropractic therapy may be required for renewal.

Score 14+: Taking time off is not a luxury—it's imperative!

I use these questions in my public speaking and over the last couple of years, the scores of my audiences have gone up dramatically. The test hasn't changed, but the increased scores indicate how starved we are as a society for a little time off and time out.

Left- and Right-Brain Functions during Stress

When we are in the midst of chaos, our right-brain functioning shuts off, and we rely solely on our left brain. Let's look at the characteristics of left-brain and right-brain function according to Daniel Murrell, MD and his article "Left brain vs. right brain: Fact and fiction" for Medical-NewsToday.com in 2018.

Left Brain	Right Brain
Language	Shapes
Linear	Holistic
Logical	Intuitive
Digital	Spatial
Abstract	Analogical
Concrete	Symbolic
Reason	Imagination
Analytical	Gestalt
Beat Music	Melody
Sequential	Sporadic
Time-bound	Timeless

Some people will be more attracted to the right-brain versus left-brain characteristics, but we need both. What happens during stress and overload is that the attributes of the right brain become inaccessible, which means we lose our intuitiveness and imagination. The way to bridge back over to our holistic right brain is to find the calm in the midst of the storm.

Choose Your Values Carefully

Once, during a Hawaiian vacation, I was in escrow to purchase a new home. I awoke one morning with gut-twisting anxiety over my realtors:

they were attempting to make additional money at my expense by steering me toward their termite contractor and mortgage people, each of whom charged a higher rate—and kicked back a finder's fee to the realtors.

During that trip, I learned about the Aloha spirit of the island; that spirit values working together without harming nature or others. I realized then how much I appreciated people who conduct their lives following this principle. I also understood why our realtors—whom I had known casually for years—looked so worn down.

Our aging process speeds up during stressful, sleepless, and frustrating times in our lives. When the *chaos tornadoes* hit hard, we need to apply damage control until they finally move on. We need to counter the aging process that kicks into gear when we advance ourselves at the cost of another or let the chaos of others rule our lives.

The symptoms of stress discussed in this chapter provide insight when you are unbalanced and have physical warning signs. If things don't change and your priorities don't shift, then illness, relationship woes, and work issues may be just around the corner. I know it's not easy to unplug, but please heed the warnings with this information at hand. You can now monitor your crisis reserve account and make healthy and life-affirming deposits. And, while you're at it, it couldn't hurt to put down your phone and disconnect from technology and reconnect to your soul.

Chapter 4
Defining Moments

Success is not final, failure is not fatal: it is the
courage to continue that counts.
~Winston S. Churchill

What is life but five to seven big events that change everything? These are defining moments that come unexpectedly to change the course of our lives. During a defining moment, we have perceptions and insights that make a permanent mark and often shape the future of our decisions.

Before the September 11, 2001, terrorist attacks on the United States, people didn't think about external chaos and stress on a regular basis. This horrific event became a collective defining moment for the world because so many lives were lost, and all the victims had done was wake up and go about their business one fine Tuesday morning.

We all have life-changing moments that are etched in our memories forever. A marriage proposal, the death of a loved one, or news of a national tragedy become markers in our lives. But there are other events, too, that are less definitive, yet have impact. A defining moment for one person can be a mere blip on the screen for someone else. One example of this is the well-known "he said, she said" phenomenon, where two people have completely different recollections of the same incident. We see this also when siblings reminisce about a shared childhood. The stories they tell of past occurrences may differ considerably. One sister may remember that Dad was always there for her, while another insists that he was never around. Or a husband and wife might vacation with another couple, and later the wife may discuss her impression of their friends' marital problems, while her husband may not have seen any rift at all.

When we compile our responses to a new situation, it is our defining moments that provide a reference point. There are as many viewpoints as there are people. Is it any wonder that communication is often a challenge? What makes defining moments unique is that our vivid impression of them often shapes the direction of our lives. These impressions become the basis for future responses, and this is how the way we rise above the chaos can define us.

The Longest Day

Some defining moments are game-changers! A defining moment that began to acquaint me with the medical world occurred when I joined my parents in Puerto Vallarta for some much-needed R and R. I thought this would be a perfect escape from the pressures of my sales job. Our hotel was right on the ocean, and the ambience immediately mellowed me into a blissful state. Unhappy as I was in my career as a food broker in the 1990's, I figured, *work is a drag, but as long as I can break away for good times like this, I can make it through.*

We toured the area and lunched in the quaint village before heading back for an afternoon swim. It was a dazzling Margaritaville sort of day, with smiling, suntanned people frolicking to the sounds of Mariachis. I became more relaxed with every breath. With the sparkling surf beckoning to us, Dad and I decided to go for a swim. As soon as we dived into the water, a set of big breakers began to roll in. Having spent many summers by the Great Lakes, body surfing was a favorite family pastime. Dad and I joyfully took on the waves, laughing and splashing, until a huge one knocked me upside down. When I finally got myself together and raised my head out of the surf, I turned around and noticed that my dad was no longer there.

As I scanned the beach, my eyes suddenly caught sight of something floating in the water about fifty yards away. *It couldn't be.* It was too shocking to comprehend. One minute I'd been in a movie-like dreamscape, the whole world warm and wonderful. *That object couldn't be my father. Not him. Not floating face down.* The adrenaline coursed through my shocked body as I half-ran, half-stumbled through the water to his side. Refusing to draw a breath of my own, I turned him over. He wasn't breathing. I felt trapped in a slow-motion nightmare, screaming for help as I pulled his six-foot body toward the shore. I kept calling out, yelling out to God and whoever else could hear me for help and divine action. Out of nowhere, a circle of people appeared, and heroic efforts were made to bring my father back to life. While someone was performing CPR, I ran toward the hotel, screaming for an ambulance, praying for a miracle.

But it wasn't to be.

One of the doctors on the beach had tested the reflexes in my father's legs, and as he suspected, a broken neck was the probable cause of his drowning. The waves sent him crashing head-first into the sand, snapping the C4 and C5 vertebras in his neck, rendering him paralyzed and utterly helpless.

Defining moments are what change the course of our lives. In one random instant, the best day of my life suddenly erupted into an explosion of pain and irreversible loss. This experience taught me that no one can be sure of anything beyond their next breath. We have no guarantee that our health will hold up, that our loved ones will escape harm, or that our world itself will remain intact. Knowing how fragile we are, and at the same time how strong, I found the courage to ultimately change my life. The final gift my father gave me as I pulled him out of the water that dreadful day was the igniting of my own power, a spiritual bequest passed from father to child.

I had always admired him. In our co-dependent relationship, I had given my power away to him in childhood. My overly protective, knows-everything dad could do no wrong. Before he left this Earth, he gave this power back to me. I believe that when an entity dies, it leaves a special essence behind. Anyone who has been privileged to witness a death can attest to learning and gaining from the experience. You cannot witness either the beginning of life nor its end and not feel a stirring in your soul.

A New Path

We never know exactly where we stand in this journey of life but defining moments can help clarify our vision. I had known that the trials in my life were helping me evolve into something more. Within a year of my father's passing, I married for the first time, a miracle in itself. I had gone through my 20's and was heading into my late 30's before I was destined to march down the aisle. What I had learned in the defining moment of my father's death was that in order to change my life, I had to *start now.* So, when my beloved proposed, I made the commitment to marry without hesitation.

Within months of my marriage, I relinquished the security of my sales position and started my own company. I began teaching others that life satisfaction is a priority, and whatever transformation we must make for this to occur is essential. Just find the *creative life solution,* I told my clients, and go for it.

Some defining moments are less dramatic than others, but every one of these realizations is significant. When we learn that a friend has betrayed us or that a relationship must end, or we discover untapped talents within ourselves, our lives are never again quite the same. Defining moments alter our perceptions, attitudes, and beliefs; defining moments shape our lives.

Staying Alive … Staying Alive

An earlier version of this work was my first book, *Staying Calm in the Midst of Chaos*, written right before the terrorist attacks of September

11, which changed our country. With a mission to bring this Stay Calm and Create Calm message to the world, I embarked on a lengthy eighteen-month book and speaking tour. After a trip to Cleveland, I found a lump in my left breast and it was stage 3 breast cancer!

With all my natural approaches to health, I didn't want to start my breast cancer treatment with a mastectomy. After all, it was the twenty-first century, and the doctors were offering me, in 2003, the exact same treatment both of my grandmothers had in the '70's. I didn't want to have chemo, surgery, and radiation. After all, I was tired from the book tour.

It only takes one thought in a defining moment to plot the course to a new life. Mine was the single idea that *I want to save my breast!* From that single quest alone, I had the courage to forgo the surgery. In our efforts to manage chaos and stress, defining moments become our repertoire of resources. We say to ourselves, *if I got through that, I can handle anything.* Healing cancer without surgery proved to be another defining moment that empowered my psyche to tackle even greater challenges. So once again, chaos was the great teacher, giving me an education that I could build from.

How Do We Reframe Violence?

After a high school shooting resulting in the deaths of several students, a memorial for the victims was televised locally. As I watched the service, I was struck by the calm demeanor of the high school principal. She was clearly holding back grief and anger, but as she spoke, her message of hope and goodness came through. She emphasized the strength of the community, people from all walks pulling together to face this tragedy. Her manner was impressive; you could feel her inner peace in the throes of chaos and tragedy.

Self-Exploration: Your Defining Moments

Have you been through a major crisis in your life when, in the midst of it all, you were able to feel a sense of calm and control? Think about the situation, describe it in detail, and consider your sources of strength. Have you been through a major ordeal where you were feeling chaotic, restless, and out of control? Describe that situation and to what you attribute your lack of power.

Defining Moments Exercise: A Crisis You Handled Calmly

Describe the situation:

Why do you think you reacted this way?

What lessons did you learn about you?

What success was gained as a result?

Defining Moments Exercise: A Crisis That Created Chaos

Describe the situation:

Why do you think you reacted this way?

What lessons did you learn about you?

What success was gained as a result?

Become a Stronger Swimmer

Let's face it ... Sometimes life just throws you into the deep end of the pool. Mary, a recent client, came to me in crisis one day. After hearing about her situation, I suggested that God wanted her to be a stronger swimmer, so he threw her into the deep end of the pool. Remember when you were learning to swim as a child? If all you did was paddle about in the shallow end where you could easily reach the bottom, then you would never know the strength of your arms and upper back to hold you up. She liked the metaphor and repeated it to me often ... it became hers.

Some people get thrown into the deep end of the pool a time or two; others practically live there. I had the joy of working with someone who lived there, a very strong swimmer indeed. In all my years of working with patients, I never met another one like Corina. She had a seven-page medical history because she had been through so many health challenges since the age of 10, including autoimmune diseases like Sjogren's syndrome and lupus, loss of hearing, loss of sight in one eye, mobility issues, digestive disorders, and sensitivity to environmental stress. She had been on a variety of medications most of her life. As if this wasn't enough of a challenge to carry, she fell backward while walking on a wet marble floor in an office building and when she hit the back of her head, she lost her voice. By the time I worked with her, she hadn't spoken a word in fifteen years! Can you even begin to imagine?

As she stood before me upon admission, her eyes twinkled. In her presence I was reminded, *rather than pray for a lighter load to carry—ask for a stronger back.* What I found when I was working with Corina was that I was in front of one of the strongest backs I'd ever met. Not only was she resilient, but she was also one of the most positive people I'd ever spent patient-advocate time with.

She was so inspiring that generous friends pooled their resources together to finance her treatment. She taught me to never give up on faith and hope.

Even in times of relative calm, we can still strengthen our swimming skills with positive thoughts and prayers that will bolster us in the face of our next challenge.

The Better I Know Myself, the Better I Show Myself

In my early life before my dad's accident, i.e. the Longest Day, I remember thinking that I wasn't quite sure who I was. I never delved inside to see if there was an original, one-of-a-kind *me* in there.

The best decision I ever made was to take the time to do this. I was in my late 20's then and without romantic distractions, so I had the time and energy to try and understand myself. During my early years of self-discovery, I met with a minister who had a busy teaching and counseling schedule. A session with Judith was like baring your soul before God. At that time, I thought I wanted to become a minister myself, and her community church seemed ideal. But it wasn't meant to be, since Judith was thinking of closing up shop in San Diego and moving to Taos. During our work together, she suggested I go on a weekend retreat and spend my time enjoying nature, listening to music, writing, and reflecting.

Of all Southern California's glorious places, I chose a mountain resort area near Palm Springs, called Idyllwild. I brought all I needed for the weekend—food, books, and music—and I checked in to a cozy little cabin. But instead of finding serenity, I became so anxious after the first night alone that I spent most of the next two days in town, shopping and making small talk with clerks. On Sunday afternoon as I prepared to leave, I realized I hadn't done much but shop and cavort around town, pretty much unable to spend time alone. The one book I read that weekend was *You Can Heal Your Life,* by Louise Hays. It was riveting. It was a calling-card experience that gave me a hopeful glimpse into my future.

As I read Ms. Hays's work and walked in the woods, I knew this was the kind of future I envisioned for myself.

As uplifted as I felt by this book and the beauty of Idyllwild, I didn't consider the weekend a success because I hadn't completed my assignment. My reason for going in the first place was to get acquainted with the essence of my spirit, but I'd hardly spent any time on my own.

Why did I feel so uncomfortable being by myself? What was I resisting? I knew I had to find out more.

So, I went back to Idyllwild. More than once. Each time I stayed at the same place, and each time I ended up spending more time solo and pursuing my quest, via journaling, reading, hiking, and sometimes just staring into the fire. My search was eventually rewarded by new insights and answers. Did I dare tell anyone how much I enjoyed just doing nothing? Just being. Just breathing. Just talking to myself and to God, and sometimes crying. My best days of self-discovery were those when I had no plans, just going with the flow, where one thing leads to the next. I would meet with serendipity when I lived this way and followed my inner source. This really is who I am at my best. Visiting this mountain resort changed my life, and I continue to go on these spiritual retreats and create them for my clients.

I know it has taken me many years of search and research, and this is just a beginning. Any time I discover a new facet of myself, I feel like I've hit the lottery. I'm not talking about the dutiful roles of parent, employee, business owner, volunteer, or student; those are external expressions. I'm talking about the qualities that make a good parent: a sense of responsibility, maturity, and patience, among others. And what makes a good entrepreneur? Vision, expertise, and knowledge. These are defining statements about our character, not just job titles.

The Best Discovery is Self-Discovery

The best real estate we own is the REAL estate within ourselves. When I know who I am, tranquility and confidence come naturally.

When I know who I am, crisis, chaos, and challenging situations can be resolved more easily. When I maintain my faith in trying times, people seem to show up out of nowhere to offer assistance.

Realize in chaos or happy times, your words are your entry point into the reality of your life. Your thoughts preface your words but listen to what you say in times of crisis and uncertainty. Do you give the world a picture of confidence? Or do your words convey a negative outlook and lack of trust? A victim mentality tends to create more chaos. When you hear yourself going in this direction, tighten your reins and pull back. Inner victims create lives of chaos; lives of rising above the chaos create inner warriors. Which course do you want to take?

As children trying to please Mom or Dad, we learn early on to satisfy others. However, a life of doing what's expected or what others dictate rarely serves our best interests. If we thrive on social situations, then perhaps that hotshot computer job isn't the best choice, no matter how proud and comfortable it makes our loved ones. Sales, customer service, or teaching might be a better fit for extroverts. We need to know what makes us happy. How else can we please ourselves if we don't know what we truly want or like?

With the shift toward finding spiritual meaning in our lives, we hear a lot about the importance of self-understanding. *To thine own self be true.* A nun named Karol Jakowski published a book called *Ten Fun Things to Do Before You Die.* Her list of must-dos included gaining insight and finding one's best self. Some can best do this by living alone for a time, for solitude has much to teach us. If you share a household, find a place where you can go off by yourself and escape from your daily routine. These are all ways we "find" ourselves.

Take time to work on these exercises. Write them in a special notebook. Date the entries so when you look through this material in years to come you gain a perspective. Even if you've done similar work before, ask yourself: *is more of me ready to be revealed?* Just as we improve our real estate and fix up our homes and property, we can always do the same within. From this reflective place, answer the self-discovery questions. What matters most is a warm-up exercise with a point.

What Matters Most?

Take the following quiz and see how you score.

Name five of the wealthiest people in the world.

Name five Heisman trophy winners.

Name five winners of the Miss America or Miss Universe title.

Name five people who have won the Nobel or Pulitzer Prize.

How about five or ten Academy Awards winners?

Other than the New York Yankees, name five World Series winning teams.

How did you do? For the categories that are easy, these are passions. With the exception of the trivia hounds out there, most of us don't remember many of yesterday's headliners. It's surprising how quickly we forget. What I've asked about aren't obscure achievements. These awards represent the best and brightest in their respective fields. But when the applause is over, awards tarnish, achievements are forgotten, and trophies are buried with their owners.

People Who Matter Most

Name three people you enjoy spending time with.

Name five people who have taught you something worthwhile.

Name five friends who have helped you during a difficult time.

List three of your favorite teachers.

Name three heroes whose stories have inspired you.

Was this quiz easier to take? Sure it was. The reason is that the people who make the greatest difference are not the ones with credentials, but the ones with compassion and concern. Those whose lives are materially focused may not understand the payoff in such work. It involves being reflective and vulnerable, and sometimes enduring emotional storms.

One of Maya Angelou's quotes reminds us, "I've learned that people will forget what you said, people will forget what you did, but people will never forget how you made them feel."

Self-Discovery Exercise

You are one of a kind. There is not another like you in this Universe. You are also the only one who will ever fully realize who you are and what your capabilities and weaknesses are, and only you will truly know the levels of every emotion you experience. For me, the key to life is in knowing myself, my talents, and my limitations, so I can better work and contribute to the world. And oh, the stress we save ourselves when we gain self-knowledge!

List your three to five most significant memories from **ages one to ten.**

What lesson(s) did you learn from this first decade?

List your most significant memories from **ages eleven to twenty.**

What lesson(s) did you learn from this decade?

List your most significant memories from **ages twenty-one to thirty.**

What lesson(s) did you learn from this decade?

List your most significant memories from **ages thirty-one to forty.**

What lesson(s) did you learn from this decade?

List your most significant memories from **ages forty-one to fifty.**

What lesson(s) did you learn from this decade?

List your most significant memories from **ages fifty-one to sixty.**

What lesson(s) did you learn from this decade?

List your most significant memories from **ages sixty-one to seventy.**

What lesson(s) did you learn from this decade?

List your most significant memories from **ages seventy-one to eighty.**

What lesson(s) did you learn from this decade?

(Complete for each decade to your current age.)
(P.S. Congratulations on living this long!)

A Check-Up from the Neck Up

Compare the two columns, quickly circling the qualities below that best describe you. There are no right or wrong answers.

Thoughtful	Impulsive
Serious	Humorous
Physical	Intellectual
Artistic	Scientific
Spiritual	Material
Self-oriented	Other-oriented
Care-giving	Loves pampering
Initiator	Observant
Personable	Standoffish
Arrogant	Modest
Confident	Insecure
Big-picture-oriented	Detail-oriented
Have firm boundaries	Tendency to be a doormat
Nature lover	City slicker
Enthusiastic	Apathetic
Happy	Depressed
Mischievous	Pious
Cautious	Risk-taker
Boring	Interesting
Shy	Outgoing
Dreamer	Doer
Resourceful	Wasteful
Engaging	Alienating
Restless	Peaceful

Kind	Mean-spirited
Type "A" Personality	Laid-back
Authentic	Phony
Leader	Follower
Goal-oriented	Fatalistic
Optimist	Pessimist
Gregarious	Solitary
Cup is Half Full	Cup is Half Empty
Well-coordinated	Klutzy
Aggressive	Passive
No-nonsense type	Whimsical

Why We Thrive—Why We Hide

After taking this quiz, we begin to see a pattern; we tend to be methodical or spontaneous, introverted or extroverted, practical or visionary, artistic or scientific. With this in mind, we can begin to see why, in certain situations or with certain people, we often thrive—or we hide. The better we know ourselves, the more we can choose situations and relationships that are in our best interests. For some, this may be just common sense, although innate wisdom is not common at all. If we have fallen into a pattern of destructive situations and relationships, we need to free ourselves from our old blueprint.

For example, if a teacher or parent implies that you aren't any good at math, science, or whatever, it often becomes a self-fulfilling prophecy. I'm not suggesting that we all have the talents of Picasso or Einstein, but I am saying we can probably complete a class or project in those areas where we were deemed unworthy and, in doing so, get a tremendous rush of self-confidence and respect.

In work relationships, are you surrounded by people who bring out your magnificence or your madness? When we connect with those who catalyze our talents, this is a lucky, blessed situation. But many will pass our way who amplify the madness. Don't crumble. Use them as a scientific test to see how much inner strength and confidence you have. In other words, don't let them take you down.

How do we release old patterns? Like all worthy ventures, it takes some doing. We must have the willingness to widen our self-perceptions, and this can be painful. If we keep hiding and avoiding challenges, we'll never realize that it's not others who limit us and cause suffering, but our own insights, biases, and ego—or lack of ego.

Changing the way we respond to stress requires us to review our priorities, and as defining moments shape our lives, we shift our perspective. Some things in life are beyond our control, but we *can* change ourselves.

Starting now.

Chapter 5
Keys to Calm

The way you see the world is the way you are going to function in it.
~Anonymous

Self-investigation takes a lot of hard work, and for most of us, that means taking a time-out. Seminar leaders, churches, and many associations put on retreats and conferences to help us find our way out of darkness and into the light of understanding and acknowledgment. Time away is a key to calmness because if you are always in a time crunch, you can't digest what life's serving up to teach you. My mantra is: *we move too fast to digest our lives.*

It's just like eating your food: you don't assume you chew a few bites and you've got all the nutrition you need. You know it takes time to assimilate the nutrition, and that's why eating slowly or not running to get second helpings is important. When we keep shoveling on those life achievements and continually pushing ourselves, we aren't assimilating the jewels and nudges life is leaving within us. If you are always in a time crunch, you may miss this aspect of life, which is what makes it all meaningful.

Through my work with others on self-investigations, I have come to realize that most stress patterns are self-inflicted. If we can unhook these old patterns of rejection, denial, betrayal, and pride, we can attain a new sense of calm and freedom. There are a number of ways of accomplishing this: in twelve-step programs, members take a personal inventory; Catholics go to confession; and, in Judaism, there are annual rituals of assessment during Yom Kippur.

Uncover, Discover, Discard

My childhood stuff surfaced in my early 30's when I was unmarried and finding it difficult to trust people. There was a popular book at the time by John Bradshaw: *Healing the Shame that Binds You*. I wanted to understand the role I played in my mid-west, high functioning alcoholic family. I was doing some serious investigating to understand my reactions to things that caused internal chaos.

I learned in working with skilled therapists that I had a severe relationship with my mother, for several reasons. First, my father adored me and showered me with attention; after all, I took after him and had a similar personality. My mother, as dutiful wives were in the 1960's, was second in command. She didn't receive quite the same recognition and adoration as my father did. Second, her hands were already full by the time I arrived on the scene. My older brother (for a myriad of reasons) needed her attention, so his developmental and emotional needs were her focus. Third, there was also tension and strain because of my father's stressful job and his place in the community. My father was an entrepreneur and president of a company, which meant my mother was a president's wife. She was like a first lady with the eyes of society on her. She had to manage her image, and the two men in my family seemed her top priority.

It's one thing not to be favored by a parent, but eventually, when I had a lifestyle change in my late 20's that involved not consuming alcohol, my drinking and foodie family made me a target of their dysfunction. As the scapegoat for all that was wrong, it seemed to me the entire tribe pretty much rejected me. Aunts, uncles, cousins, and nieces all made it clear, by not inviting me to or informing me of weddings or funerals, that they weren't friendly toward me.

As an adult, when I tried to unravel what happened, I found two possible reasons for my disregard by the family: A) I left the mid-west and moved to California as quickly as I could after college and got a new lifestyle or B) The family needed a scapegoat, someone who all could agree was the "black sheep." For those not familiar with this dynamic, the black sheep is an outcast and outlet for the darkness in a family. Regardless of whichever reason was the cause of this lack of respect or acknowledgment from my family, the treatment continued well into adulthood and mid-life as I continued to build a business, write books, and be featured on TV.

Friends or Teachers?

Eventually, I found ways to replace the need for my blood family and to heal my ensuing anger, because blaming your family or others is a pointless way to live. No one is perfect, and we all have something to learn from our family members; they are our most insightful teachers.

I always resonated with the idea that there are two categories of people: not friends and enemies, but instead, friends and "teachers." Your friends love and support you through good times and bad. Your "teachers," on the other hand, point out your areas of weakness through a lack of support, criticism, or even rejection. The point is this: We have no enemies. When we think of those who betray, deceive, and manipulate us not as enemies but as *teachers*, we can overcome resentment and anger. This is a wonderful philosophical way to transform hurtful wounds into something powerful and healing. If I think I'm having a bad day because more than three "teachers" have appeared to point out my limitations, chances are the problem has to do with my perceptions, and I should be looking in the mirror rather than casting blame.

Judging Versus Compassion

When we're face-to-face with judgment, we can go down the road of self-doubt and despair, but there are other options. Instead of letting judging and menacing types break our spirits, we can choose to grow. To see these perceived attacks as a motivation for change. If we react with constant fear, blame, or judgment in return, we can create a spiritual "dis-ease" within ourselves. If someone is judging you as "less than" and you start judging them as an egomaniac, then you are as much at fault as they are. The continuous judgment of others alienates us and causes a spiritual malady.

I once had a patient who was a successful entrepreneur going around the country teaching people how to buy homes and get rich. At the beginning of the relationship, he wanted to work with me; he bought all my books and showed interest and intrigue in my story of healing cancer.

Once he got everything figured out at the hospital, he moved up and no longer needed a patient advocate. He made it clear he no longer *had time for me* because whatever services I was useful for, he'd already gotten. So even with cancer in his body, he kept his strong *I'm-in-charge* personality up front.

I eventually learned compassion for people who can't lighten up a bit while they are conquering illness. I was taught by the doctors and nurses how to let go of the insults or rejections. All I know is that when chaos arrives, we learn so much when we shift our perspective. One of my favorite approaches to offset difficult people and situations is to say to the experience: *what strength can I learn here for myself?*

Today's Trial Can Heal Yesterday's Pain

Until these issues of judging, blaming, or being a victim are resolved, we will often recreate scenarios to know where we stand and how repaired we are from life's scars. I have always looked at life as a classroom, and each encounter is here to teach us where we stand in the life lessons we are here to learn. I know it sounds simple, but it does offer relief if you don't like the "lesson plan" lately for your life.

I was working with a cancer patient who discussed her family issues often as part of her cancer treatment. Sarah was a kind-hearted soul who wanted to connect with everyone, and she did so easily. Her cancer healing was a success, but she was having secondary problems and getting tired of being sick and unable to live a normal life. Then one day, Sarah arrived at the hospital all out of sorts. Instead of charming the place, she was in full-on self-pity mode. I offered to work with her, and on the way to treatment, she told me that her husband had vented his frustrations about having a wife who was sick for so long and the resulting financial hardship. I could see she felt unappreciated and scared.

I suggested she spend her visit at the hospital recuperating from her health issues and from her anger at her husband's upsetting comments. If she could see how being a victim to others' opinions had been an old pattern, she could untangle it within her soul.

I advised her to gather her strength and self-belief and use them to stop viewing her husband's angry words as a personal attack but rather as an opportunity for growth. And once she felt stronger and empowered again, she could correct this matter with an adult conversation, reminding him what a gem of a wife she was. It was important to see that her trial by cancer and subsequent healing provided a life lesson plan for them both to rise above the chaos. They both had lessons to learn, and together they could come out stronger and closer than before cancer.

It's a shift to gratitude that makes all the difference, because chaos is the great teacher. So, if you are going through turmoil in your life right now, stop to say thank you; challenges like these sharpen your skills and wits.

Adverse Childhood Experience

Self-investigation won't happen, for most of us, until the pain in our lives is too much to bear. I didn't learn about adverse childhood experiences (ACEs) research until after I went through my self-investiga-tion and soul reconstruction. According to the website *www.samhsa.gov* and their article "Adverse Childhood Experiences" in 2018, ACEs "are stressful or traumatic events, including abuse and neglect." Once I started looking at the ACEs research on those who had endured extreme child-hood chaos and trauma, I was so grateful. It explained a lot about my life and my family's dysfunction and neglect. There were so many insights on the accompanying health challenges adults with ACE backgrounds face, including substance abuse issues.

In 2017, there was research called "Methods to Assess Adverse Child-hood Experiences of Children and Families: Toward Approaches to Pro-mote Child Well-being in Policy and Practice" by Dr. Bethell, in *US National Library of Medicine*, that stated, "Although important variations exist, available ACEs measurement methods are similar and show con-sistent associations with poorer health outcomes in absence of protective factors and resilience."

The paradigm-shifting neurobiological and epidemiologic findings show cumulative, cascading, and multidimensional effects of trauma and stress associated with ACEs. ACEs include physical or emotional abuse or neglect, loss of a parent, family discord and divorce, exposure to alco-hol or drug abuse, mental illness in the home, or violence in the home or neighborhood. The high prevalence of ACEs in the child and adult pop-ulation combined with evidence of their effect on health, life satisfaction, and social and medical care costs have now positioned ACEs as a matter of public health in the United States as well as globally. In the article, the focus was on the measurement of ACEs of children and families in research, public health, and clinical practice.

When I observed how difficult this situation was for Sarah, I intu-itively knew it was more than a hurtful, husband-and-wife exchange of words. I could sense that something was coming up from her childhood that needed to be energetically and emotionally healed. For those who have had adverse childhood experiences, it takes years of soul searching to grasp how profoundly these childhood patterns of pain and trauma affect our adult lives and call out to be healed.

I identify with Sarah's story because I, like so many of us, have had this kind of experience of wanting others to be kind, approve of us, and like us one hundred percent of the time. However, it's during challenging times that we need to take the focus off others and heal our wounds or childhood traumas. It's only once we learn to be less reliant on others and gain self-reliance that we evolve enough to overcome our old childhood scripts of low self-esteem or self-worth.

A Friend and Mentor

I was 28 years old when I met him. Ken was a 70-year-old man who had quit drinking a decade earlier and devoted his life to spiritual studies and practices. I loved to be around him, for he exuded a kind of calm that I could feel just walking into his home. He loved God. One of his favorite books was *Practicing the Presence* by Joel Goldsmith. I felt the Presence when I was with Ken. Sadly, our time together was too short. We had one year as the best of friends, and in some ways, he was my first patient, because that last year of his life I cooked for him regularly as he taught me esoteric truths that I still carry within my heart today. One of my favorite sayings of his was, "Character defects aren't the real you; they are like barnacles on the bottom of a ship. Remove the barnacles and your ship will be ready for smooth sailing." Since he passed through my life, this phrase has guided my healing help as a people developer and patient advocate. It's a key to remaining calm in the midst of the most turbulent storms because it speaks to getting rid of the false self, letting go of the façade we all put on to get through life. One day you won't need that façade because you will have discovered the true you. That is what we are doing when we look at our internal chaos and the self-inflicted habits or mechanisms that overwhelm us.

How to Use Journaling to Reduce Stress

Some of you might laugh when I suggest that you write about the things that are stressing you. The idea that there is any time to write about the problems of an over-scheduled life seems absurd. I used to always dial up my friends to discuss my latest upset rather than taking the time to sit down and write about it. Then one day, I heard the "magic formula," and I learned why writing this "stuff" out is such good therapy.

I was at a conference in Hawaii, and a speaker explained that when we talk about our problems, we engage about 100,000 nerve cells in the process. But when we put our thoughts on paper, we activate something like 2,000,000 cells! The combination of visual and manual processes engages the brain twenty times more than mere lip service.

One of my long-time clients was a computer engineer who always scheduled the time to attend the "Day of Healing" seminars I hosted for my clients. She talked about her system to inventory her various stressors. Being an engineer, it was a very methodical but effective process that I've used with countless clients. She decided to use a page in her journal and draw a line dividing it in half so she could separate external from internal pressures. Her list looked something like this:

External Stress	Internal Stress
Being a Single Parent	Unresolved Relationship Issues
Job Change	Financial Worries
Uncomfortable Living Conditions	Feelings of Insecurity
Legal Entanglements	Desire to Leave Past Behind
Unfriendly Neighbors	Yearning for a Gentler Way of Life

This simple exercise helps put our problems into focus. Most of the things in the left column are beyond our control. The items on the right, however, describe the way we *feel* about the pressures in our lives, and that is something we *can* change. Just writing down and acknowledging what our stressors are is a positive action toward gaining serenity. If you can also share your concerns with a trusted friend, it makes your load even less of a burden.

See if this formula works for you. Remember, it's the items on the right you want to rewire in your brain.

Unloading Our Baggage

Sometimes we need to revisit the past to relieve ourselves of stress we are carrying around from too many unpleasant or traumatic yesterdays. When we are coping with any kind of loss, we often muscle our way through until the pain diminishes or the situation and feelings begin to shift. However, by coping this way, we don't fully experience our emotional upheavals, and they never fully leave us. We continue to reference *that marriage*, *that year*, or *that job* with distress because we haven't healed our perspective of the situation.

If you keep accumulating these unresolved issues, you end up carrying an elephant-sized load. You don't know why you've lost your zest for life. You might remember feeling freer when you were younger, and you begin to lament your lost youth. But guess what? You haven't lost your youth; you've just lost touch with the light-hearted joys of an earlier time.

Understanding our emotional patterns can help us in navigating a calmer life. Getting calmer is the first step to rising above the chaos. Let's say you're someone who always has to be number one. You are uncomfortable at meetings or social events where someone else is in the limelight. A great way to gain a new perspective is to purposefully attend an event as an observer or allow someone else to control the evening. If you feel you're wasting your time when you are *not* the guest of honor, ask yourself why you always need the spotlight. What part of you has this driving need for attention? Can you find some value in situations without crowds, applause, and attention? Can you still love yourself when you're not number one?

Lightening up and releasing these painful accumulations makes us more open to what life has to offer. Opportunities come our way when we are receptive, and trust me, colleagues, friends, and loved ones can sense when we are walled off by old baggage. If we learn to release this inner chaos, we can then walk into a business meeting, a party, or an annual event and share our lightness with the world. We are the calm in the midst of chaos. People want to know us, they want to hire us, and they want to love us.

The Body Knows

When we start to retrace these painful accumulations called "energy cysts" (i.e. blocks) and allow them to leave us mentally, emotionally, and spiritually, that is the moment we become lighter and more youthful. I call this process *healing,* and this is exactly the process that shifted my own life from one of upheaval to one of joy.

Before my work as a patient advocate, I had a private practice as a craniosacral therapist. These were the years that prepared me for executive coaching and working with those healing from cancer. One of my clients was a financial planner who had multiple sclerosis as well as other health problems. She kept going to doctors who treated her symptoms surgically. She was cut up like a patchwork quilt from operations on her stomach, pancreas, and gallbladder. The procedures were performed because her organs were shutting down. During our session, I saw that her heart was clearly blocked. I dialogued with her, and finally said, "When did you put a shield around your heart?"

Startled, she replied, "My mother died when I was 10, and as we buried her, I told myself I never wanted to love anyone again. I felt if I loved someone, they would leave me."

I told her, "Your internal organs are shutting down because you've cut yourself off from love. We need love to survive. Love fuels every cell and system in our bodies." Her body was deteriorating, and she was "dying" from this lack of love and trust.

Through her tears, she murmured, "I just can't let someone in and let myself be loved."

I smiled. "It's too late; I've been loving you since the moment you came in here today."

Suddenly, her body began to respond. As this block was lifted from her heart, her organs started to reactivate. It sounded like a symphony. The stomach played, then the spleen, then the pancreas, liver, and intestines. It was the most amazing orchestra of healing as all these organs were set in motion and began to play. It was the music of healing I heard that day.

It is common for those who have unhealed grief to try and shield their heart. The problem is that many of us leave the shield in place for the rest of our lives and never fully open our hearts to love. Heart shields are like armor and can be the origin of heart disease if a person keeps that love and hurt bottled inside.

If we take in each past or present experience that seemed like trauma or an upset and we look at it with awe and wonder, we might learn something. By doing this, we are asking our hearts for answers, not our minds. Wondering is a receptive and peaceful approach to problem resolving. It opens us up to answers.

The Wonder Approach

Years before my diagnosis, I wondered why breast cancer was an epidemic. Just putting that question out into the Universe, I found research on how antiperspirants were blocking the normal function of sweat glands. This could be a problem of toxins not being released around the lymph nodes and sweat glands. Based on research from a prominent cancer agency, I found that the normal function of sweat glands was impaired by the aluminum-based compounds that are the active ingredients in antiperspirants. They block the sweat glands to keep sweat from getting to the skin's surface. Some research has suggested that these aluminum compounds may be absorbed by the skin and cause changes in estrogen receptors of breast cells. Sure enough, in my mind, I asked, and an answer came. I found this helpful, when perplexing matters presented themselves after that, I would use the wonder approach.

Does Money Mean You're Better?

Another incident cropped up one day, as I wondered about the sequences of my financial life. Suddenly, there it was, an answer to my question: *why aren't I rich?* The answer came to me via a complaint from a wealthy lady *I'd never met*, who was using her influence, money, and superiority to scar my reputation. It was a terribly frustrating situation that made me grateful I hadn't chose making money and pushing others around as a sport.

Wondering is posing a question to the Universe to help you rise above the chaos of your situation and to provide a significant key to calm. I am grateful that many times I've wondered about my childhood and a variety of life experiences, and I've gotten an answer.

Whether you decide to adopt the wonder approach, journaling, a twelve-step program, or talking with a mentor or therapist, there are keys to finding calm in even the most trying of times. Often, it's a mind shift from *why is this happening to me* to *what can I learn from this?* This might be recognition of childhood traumas or an acknowledgment of toxic relationships. And it's a shift toward gratitude and thanking the great teachers in our lives—even if those lessons were hard-won. It's a mind shift that promotes healing by looking at our baggage and then letting it go.

Chapter 6

Life Transitions Reset Our Priorities

Any transition is easier if you believe in yourself and your talent.
~Priyanka Chopra

There is one guarantee in life: constant change. You can fight and kick against the currents of change, but the effort is futile. Life is continuously evolving, from a cellular level to a spiritual level, and part of taming the chaos in your life is learning to make peace with the process. If you're an ambitious grow-getter, expect even more transitions. Even people who aren't here to become a senator or climb Mount Everest are going to experience personal and professional opportunities for growth. It's part of life and what it means to be alive, as we mark moving from childhood to holding our children and then grandchildren, with transitions galore in between.

Transitions cause chaos because, for those who choose to grow through their tragedies, there is a necessary reset to your priorities. I've observed in my own life that every time I take a bold step forward, some little surprise by the name of "two steps back" is waiting around the bend. Is it testing me to see if I really want another book tour or best friend?

Why can't that climb to success come without blisters? In the midst of chaos, we all ponder and process these things.

We are often tested the most when our business or personal relationships transition, which is why the last chapter of this book deals with relationships and trusting the process. As my life lesson plan has taught me: with growth comes setbacks. If we can embrace setbacks as set*ups*, we can rise more easily. If I release someone or something from my life that isn't working out, I then allow a space for something great to come in.

Neutralizing the Stress of Transitions

My husband and I were traveling on a long-awaited vacation. This was a restorative family vacation, as my husband Bryan had just been through a major grocery-store buy-out for a company he had worked in for over fifteen years. The buy-out news wasn't made available until the ink had dried and all federal regulations been met. However, nine months before the announcement, all the policies and rules in his work environment had changed. As a supervisor, he had to comply with and enforce the new rules without explanation.

This was a difficult situation. I had never seen him faced with so many stressors without knowing why. Some transitions are far out of our hands, and can even be hidden, yet we absolutely know that we are in the midst of one. The day the announcement was made that Amazon bought Whole Foods, we let out a huge sigh of relief in our household. We felt that all the changes Amazon wanted had already been put in place as part of the acquisition. Fortunately for our family, it all worked out.

On the first leg of our trip to Yellowstone National Park, we stayed just one hour north of Las Vegas in a small town named Eureka. I was excited for the two weeks ahead, so I awoke early to work out in the gym. Funny how life shows up to confirm how important each step of survival is. While in the gym, I meet a 30-something technology executive from Spain. As we started to chat around seven o'clock, I learned he was visiting the United States for a business conference in Las Vegas. I asked him why he was not in Viva Las Vegas enjoying all the city has to offer. He told me he was meeting up for a day of sightseeing at Bryce Canyon with his work buddy from Germany.

These IT executives both planned a day in nature, hiking and exploring, before attending their conference. I was so impressed. Here two international technology guys, who worked seventy-five-hour work weeks, were traveling to nature to spend a day together before their intensive Las Vegas conference. We were delighted that our paths had crossed, as our mutual missions were to absorb nature's beauty to offset stress.

Finding YOUR Fix

Many high-performance and ultra-successful people just can't seem to push the pause button and get a nature or relaxation reset. However, your ultimate success depends upon it. Embracing the need for life balance in a transition time makes the future easier to discern. For some people, the fix is as simple as rest.

As we all know, one of the greatest inventors of the twentieth century was Thomas Edison. The inventor of the light bulb and many other patents had a great way of problem solving which I love. His approach to solving scientific problems was ... taking a nap. He trusted rest as the vehicle to get him from point A to point B. Going from point A to B is exactly what transitioning is.

Many of the corporate and international executives I've worked with have found it challenging to find a space for self—a common theme in this book. The more promotions they are given, the harder it is to access downtime. Especially with international executives, the job is endless; they can work around the clock. But finding your fix to get your brain and body on track should be everyone's goal. Studying the genius pioneers of the twentieth century can garner some clues; companies now have pods for relaxation that harken back to the strategies of Edison. It's imperative that our minds, bodies, and souls have a respite during times of transition. This is so vital. If you refuse to unplug, the stress and chaos can become overwhelming. Learning to lean into rest and relaxation is a life skill and minimizes the confusion that can come during ending and beginning times.

Reset Yourself

One of my clients, Lily, was making a career transition because she knew the company that she was working for was not setting up her (or her team) for success. After plenty of pressure from the upper executives and a sense that nothing was ever going to be enough to please her boss, she decided to terminate the contract.

Even when you know all the signs are pointing toward the exit, there is still trepidation in your soul. Lily liked the high-level salary and accomplishments, which were her top priority. But once their poor treatment began to wear her down, the importance of her cherished VP career changed. She now wanted peace of mind.

I reminded Lily that she *needed* to reset herself to make this change. Then I suggested she journal and mark her progress in her final thirty days on the exit ramp.

If you're in a transition and need to redefine your life priorities, here is an exercise I highly recommend to help you move the situation forward. You already have the understanding that you're going to be making a major change, so begin to make time deposits into the new endeavor you are about to pursue. This is helpful even if you don't have a game plan for where you're heading. You just have clarity that you need to exit where you've been.

Time-Deposit Exercise

Wake up thirty minutes early each day of the final thirty days of your job (or whatever you are exiting). Use this activity as preparation for whatever new experience is coming your way. Grab a journal or notepad and date the page with your countdown numbers: Day 30, 29, 28, and so on until your last day.

Next, get quiet and breathe. Think about this transition and where you want to be on the other side of it. Write out a task list or your desires for the day. Write a little love note to yourself. Focus on your confidence to find your way, start anew, and help yourself get up on your feet.

WHATEVER you are staring down, it's time to set your intention and move forward. When I'm transitioning, I waffle. *Can I really survive life without this title, person, or endeavor?* Of course, the answer is yes! Reinvention revitalizes the soul. New beginnings wake up the brain cells. If unresolved emotional baggage is present, there will likely be some restless agitation as well. Even if emotional baggage has been resolved, this is a time when self-doubts can flare up; it's just part of the transition process.

The time-deposit exercise is helpful because you are in a situation where you are juggling two realities at once. One reality is you're moving out of a job, city, or relationship, so you have a sense of loss as endings are at hand. Pay attention to your closure messages and meanings. The second reality is the new life to come, and in your journaling, you get to imagine how life will be when the transition is complete and the new role has begun. This is an experience with lots of emotions and ideas swirling, from reluctant trepidation to excited anticipation. Even when the decision is made, you are saying goodbye and hello simultaneously, each and every day. This unique scenario is why the thirty-day journal exercise is so grounding.

Create Your Own "One Page"

The work of Charles Hobbs, a time management guru in the 1980's, focused on identifying life values and priorities. His work with implementing time management tactics was adopted by Daytimers™, who partnered with Hobbs in teaching his programs to corporate clients.

Every one of us can benefit from learning these valuable techniques. According to Hobbs's philosophy, the first step in managing one's time is to identify life values and priorities, which he calls *unifying principles*. Once you affirm them, you then schedule your time with respect to those values and goals. In his book *Time Power*, Hobbs states, "If you know what you want to achieve and you schedule your time to accommodate your goal, you will accomplish it."

I was impressed with Hobbs's approach to time and recognized that his philosophy was critical to helping people stay focused during transitions.

Because of the various tools I use to help people gain clarity during transition times, I often use the unifying principles exercise during corporate trainings. It is always a favorite to get people relaxed and ready to learn. Most of us enjoy telling others what we stand for, if given a chance.

If you decide to follow Hobbs's lead, don't just *think* about your values and priorities. Tattoo them on your arm—or at least jot them down in ink. When it comes to our dreams, goals, and priorities, we need to be definitive. Writing them down is a contract we make with ourselves. We then create a permanent record to refer to when we start to waffle, and that in itself is an essential step toward attaining our goals.

What would be on your One Page? How could you use your unifying principles to more effectively and efficiently transition through life? Think of these unifying principles as the foundation for living a more satisfying life. When I look at my unifying principles, I see the themes of family, personal integrity, healthy lifestyle, and spiritual growth. These are the core values that I use as a guide for living and especially as a way to ground myself in the most chaotic of times.

Now it's your turn: Ready! Set! Go!

Write down what YOU stand for:

MY Unifying Principles:

1._____

_____

2._____

_____

3._____

_____

4._____

_____

5._____

_____

6._____

_____

7._____

_____

8._____

_____

The New Year is a Useful Transition Time

When experiencing life transitions, we are in a time of self- and life assessments. This is especially true at the launch of a new project or new year. My ritual at the end of each year is to review the highlights reel of that year and track the highs and lows. Just looking at each quarter with personal and professional highs and lows lets me know when and where I need to make changes. I don't set my intentions for the new year until I've done the highlights reel of the old. We can do this regarding any situation: review the relationship or job highlights reel.

Just like the IT executive I met at the gym, I still get away at the end of each year to catch up with my soul. For decades I've facilitated personal and team executive retreats for those who are seeking this guidance and assistance.

Now we are about to launch into the practical tools on eating, exercise, and restoring yourself during epic challenges. The techniques offered can help you find peace during life's hardest transitions. I hope you've come to respect chaos as the great teacher and to appreciate that hard times often bring the most lasting and positive changes into our lives.

Chapter 7
Why Do We Fight Eating Right?

Let food be thy medicine and medicine be thy food.
~Hippocrates

How we fuel our bodies is always essential, but in times of high stress, it is critical. And yet it's when we're under pressure with several categories of chaos or a significant life transition that we're most likely to resort to fast foods and sweets or some other self-sabotaging behavior. However, when we are beset with adversities, these high-performance situations are when we need a diet that's like rocket fuel. That rocket fuel is simple, natural, and nutritious foods: fruits, vegetables, meats if you choose, grains, legumes, and nuts.

The more food is processed, the more it's depleted of nutrition. We need the fully fortified natural foods to deliver vitamins and minerals in an easily assimilated form. Ideally, eighty to ninety percent of our diet should come from natural foods because our bodies are designed to digest them in their fundamental form. Refined or highly-processed foods often dump sugar into the bloodstream too quickly, and the result can be fluctuating insulin levels that further stress our bodies and affect our mood and energy.

Going Natural

If you're currently living on a diet of fast food and pizza, you can start with maybe thirty- to fifty-percent natural foods and you'll soon begin to feel increased energy and well-being. Whatever enables you to function at a high level and live comfortably should be your goal. In time, you may wish to increase your natural food intake to an ideal of eighty to ninety percent.

My life experience with finding the right way to eat happened over years. I like to suggest that people be kind and encouraging to themselves when implementing new eating patterns. There is a line I've repeated several times through the years, and it's from the movie *The Natural*, starring Robert Redford as a baseball pro making a comeback after some major chaos to his pitching arm. He said, *"There's the life you learn from, and the one you live after that."*

Food Addiction: A Family Disease

My father's side of the family tended toward obesity. When I was growing up, people commented on my appetite for sweets and also on my cooking skills. I clearly had my dad's genes when it came to food. However, early on I knew I wanted to avoid looking like my 200-pound aunt or 300-pound grandmother. My fear of becoming obese became a driving force in my life. I knew I had to do something about my eating habits because I kept gaining and losing the same thirty-plus pounds over and over.

My weakness was sweets; candy and desserts were an escape from life's problems and disappointments. In an attempt to find a solution to my fluctuating weight situation, I considered a food plan that had no sugar, wheat, or flour. Had I heard about this at any other time, I might not have given it a second thought. But I was eight years into transforming my life so I could help others with ministerial studies and was getting my massage license. Suddenly some emotional baggage came up to be healed, but before I could address it, food had become my new drug of choice. Once again, I was off and running on eating binges and, at the same time, obsessing over trying to stay thin.

In my mid-30's I reached a pinnacle crisis—feeling lost in my career and single life—that I attempted to resolve with food. It was a month of popcorn, flavored coffees, and sugar-free frozen yogurt that left me feeling crazy. In the midst of this binge, I was very angry with God. I yelled and screamed at Him or Her that I had changed my life so completely for the good, yet here I was a "bleeping" mess. As the apostle Paul once wrote, "You are never closer to God then when you are angry with Him."

It was during this rage that I heard about a book that would change my life. *Food Addiction: The Body Knows*, by Kay Sheppard, introduced me to the idea of abstaining from sugar, just as I did with alcohol, which contains sugar. The book also mentioned that wheat and flour might be a problem as well, and it suggested eliminating these three items. However, that was easier said than done

In my wildest dreams, I never imagined having to relinquish all the foods that contain these ingredients to stabilize my body, mind, and spirit. But for me, that turned out to be the solution. For the first time in my life, my body weight stabilized, and no longer did I have to fear the scale galloping toward the 200 mark. Nor did I even have to worry about regaining those on-again, off-again thirty pounds.

When We Commit to Healthy Changes ... Chaos Can Arise

As soon as I committed to a healthier diet and began living on a higher plane, I found myself tested once again. Did I mention my career at the time? I worked in the food industry for twenty years and spent the later years as a food broker in sales and marketing. My clients were quality manufacturers such as Stouffer's, Nestlé, and Uncle Ben's. After I began abstaining from sugar, wheat, and flour, I continued to sell those foods, without consuming any of them.

But I did my job well. My boss was so pleased with my performance that he wanted to show his appreciation. Mars, Incorporated owned Uncle Ben's, and as a reward for doing a good job, Uncle Ben's gave us a new line to represent: Ethel M chocolates. This gourmet line of confections is made in Las Vegas, and it was a spin-off from the Mars fortune. Ethel was the mother of the clan, and hence Ethel M chocolates became the new kid on the upscale-candy block. My boss said, "Carolyn, I'd like you to be the account manager for Ethel M. Congratulations!"

Here I am, nine months off all forms of sugar, and I was about to represent a world-class chocolate line. Within days, Federal Express delivered two large boxes filled with forty pounds of mouth-watering samples to get me acquainted with the product. Resisting occasional temptation is one thing but living on an intimate basis with thought-I'd-died-and-gone-to-heaven-caliber truffles is something else. I panicked.

How could I not succumb to temptation? Where could I possibly hide these seductive morsels, so they'd be out of sight *and* out of mind? As dragon-sized doubts raced through my brain, I opened the front hall closet and placed all forty pounds of chocolate inside and slammed the door.

Then I sat in my living room wondering, *where am I going to get the strength to open these boxes and not eat myself silly?* Suddenly, I had a vision of my 300-pound grandmother. I began to recall a voice from my childhood, when my grandmother would tell us, "If you want some goodies, go to the front hall closet."

Grandmother had such a sweet tooth that she actually bribed the bakery men at her local grocery store. Entenmann's and Awrey Bakeries trucks would deliver to her home during their weekly runs because her consumption and tips made it worth their while. When the racks of goodies arrived, she had them stored in her front hall closet where she kept her stash. Strength somehow came to me through this recollection. *Don't let history repeat itself,* I told myself over and over.

I never did sample a single chocolate during my tenure as a food broker, nor have I since. I don't take full credit for this, for I believe we are given strength in times like this by a Benevolent Force or Higher Power.

Processed Food Facts

When I was still working as a food broker, I was in a position to see firsthand how many hidden ingredients are used to enhance the flavor and shelf life of processed foods. For example, plain frozen chicken breasts are usually injected with a salt solution to add flavor. If the chicken is seasoned, it likely contains more than one form of sugar and salt in addition to the injected ingredients. It's because sugar and salt appeal to our taste buds that you'll find them in almost every prepared product on the shelf. But, while excess is unhealthy, the natural sugars in fruits and grains are a source of energy, and the salts that occur naturally in vegetables, such as high-sodium celery, are essential for keeping our body's electrolytes in balance.

Getting the White Out

All the nutritionists I've interviewed believe that a healthy diet is one that is relatively free of white sugar and white flour. Some say eliminate all "whites," and that includes dairy foods as well. Why are the experts so down on these popular foods? One reason is that sugar robs the body of its natural calcium, provides no nutrition through its high-calorie content, and stimulates the pancreas so that insulin is dumped into the bloodstream, causing blood sugar levels to fluctuate out of balance. In my book co-authored by Geronimo Rubio, MD, titled *Breaking the Cancer Code*, Dr. Rubio explains that his research shows that "cancer cells are nourished by sugars and nutrients that rotate to the right side. If you have any mutating cells forming they get fed by this non-nutritional experience."

While dairy products are touted as a good source of calcium, their lactic acid content can leach calcium from the bone, canceling out the benefit. In spite of the ubiquitous "milk does a body good" ads, milk is considered by many to be unnecessary after the first year of life. Cows have four stomachs, and even they can't digest it. In the study called "Hormones in Dairy Foods and Their Impact on Public Health" it states most dairy products contain high levels of hormones, which may be carcinogenic and could affect our hormonal balance. In the Article *Does Milk Cause Cancer?* on drweil.com, scientist Ganmaa Davaasambuu, MD, PhD noted that ingestion of the estrogen present in natural milk from cows (particularly from pregnant cows) may be linked to breast, prostate, and testicular cancers in humans.

While calcium and dairy can lower the risk of osteoporosis and colon cancer, high intake can increase the risk of prostate cancer and possibly ovarian cancer. Plus, dairy products can be high in saturated fat as well as retinol (vitamin A), which at high levels can, paradoxically, weaken bones. So, obviously, nutrition studies can get confusing.

In her report, Dr. Davaasambuu cited a study comparing the diet and cancer rates in forty-two countries that showed a strong correlation between milk and cheese consumption in cancer patients. The incidence of testicular cancer among men age 20 to 39 was highest in high-consuming countries such as Switzerland and Denmark and low in Algeria and other parts of the world where people eat less dairy. She also linked rising rates of dairy consumption to the increased death rates from prostate cancer (from near zero per 100,000 men five decades ago to seven per 100,000 men today) and noted that breast cancer also appears to be linked to milk and cheese consumption.

If these things concern you, you may want to eat calcium-rich foods such as salmon and broccoli and take a good, readily-absorbed supplement. Or, if you insist on having some dairy in your diet, there are a number of organic or hormone-free brands on the market. Your local health food store is the place to find these organic dairy products. And don't forget that oat, almond, or rice milk can be a great hormone-free alternative.

Don't Forget the Fine Print

Of all the reading you do on the subject of food, labels may be the most important. Before you toss an item into your shopping cart, take time to check out its fat and sugar content as well as its list of ingredients. The words you can't pronounce are usually the preservatives and chemical additives. We know that stress alone affects hormones, sleep patterns, and energy levels. If we fuel our bodies with lots of highly-processed foods, we only intensify the problem.

Coronary heart disease is our nation's leading cause of death. We all know people who, having survived a first heart attack, are told to change their habits, particularly with regard to eating less salt and saturated fats. But you need to beware of labels that boast "no salt added" or "less fat" or "reduced calories." These big-print claims are meant to attract those seeking healthy foods, but all too often such statements, while technically accurate, are misleading.

For example, in a glass of "2%-fat" milk (98% fat-free), about one-third of the calories are derived from fat. That's a far cry from something that is truly fat-free. And "no salt added" products may still contain high levels of sodium. Forget the hype on the front of the can or package and read the small print on the back. You may wish to set your own limits, but a good guideline is three or less fat grams and under 200 grams of sodium per serving.

You Don't Have to Go It Alone

A friend of mine in the food business had a heart attack when he was only 50 years old. He dearly loved his wife and 12-year-old daughter, so he was strongly motivated to change his life. His doctor recommended a low-fat diet with lots of fruits and vegetables. John was diligent, and within six months he lost about thirty pounds and looked a decade younger. He considered himself a saved man and told everyone how wonderful he felt.

Unfortunately, this is not the end of the story. A few years later, I ran into John again and saw immediately that he had gone back to his old eating habits—lots of high fat and refined foods. All the weight returned, and that healthy, revitalized glow was just a memory. When we chatted, he told me, "I'm disgusted with myself. I hate what I'm doing, but I've got such a sweet tooth." Once John started eating occasional desserts, his new eating plan went right down the tubes.

When someone who's had such a dramatic wake-up call can't manage to stay on a healthy course, there is usually an emotional issue or attachment to food that needs to be addressed. Experts refer to this as an eating disorder, and therapy groups, one-on-one counseling, and organizations such as WW (formerly Weight Watchers) have proven highly effective for millions with this kind of problem. Twelve-step programs (which operate on an anonymous, donation-only basis) help those with food addictions (or any addiction) by providing spiritual solutions and fellowship with like-minded people. I know first-hand how powerful these programs can be to sustain people during difficult times.

If people feel the chaos in their life is driven by food, I like to encourage them. I spent decades of my life dieting in one fashion or another, until I finally realized—just as I'd always heard—*diets don't work*. You have to make a lifestyle change, and it must be one you can live with. But for a long time, I couldn't quite figure out exactly what this meant. Once I grasped the concept, it became one of my passions, and this enthusiasm helped me become more effective in all aspects of my life.

I don't recommend that everyone abstain from sugar, wheat, and flour to better manage stress. However, if you find yourself craving foods like cookies, muffins, pizza, and ice cream, and if these indulgences leave you feeling lethargic or depressed, you may want to consider a lifestyle change as disciplined as mine. Before I made that change, when

I started eating certain foods, I had to finish the whole package to be satisfied. For decades now, that hasn't been the case. Of all the goals I have achieved in my life, living in a normal-sized body day after day is one of my biggest accomplishments.

Nutritionally Dense Foods vs. Empty Calories

For most people, getting the proper balance of natural foods and keeping the empty-calorie processed stuff to a minimum will provide a buffer against stress and protection against illness.

An interesting article titled "The Original Renewable Energy Source" on the Federal Occupational Health website (https://foh.psc.gov/calendar/nutrition.html) states you can "get the most out of your calories by eating nutritionally dense food. These foods are relatively low in calories, but high in nutrition, so they can help you maintain a healthy weight while giving you a good dose of vitamins, minerals, protein, and fiber." Dense food is of course fruits and vegetables, whole grains, lean sources of protein (lean meat, seafood, soy products, eggs, beans, and nuts), and calcium-rich foods.

Our bodies are like machines, and modern medicine notwithstanding, this is one vehicle we won't be replacing any time soon. So, give yourself a minute and consider what kind of fuel you're using to get through this once-in-a-lifetime journey. Are you pampering yourself like a pricy new Lexus, or are you allowing yourself to run on empty?

The Fuel Test

Answer the following questions with a yes or no.

1. I usually eat three to five serving of fruits and vegetables every day.

    Yes_____   No_____

2. I usually refrain from junk or snack foods I'm craving.

    Yes_____   No_____

3. I eat a variety of foods each week, and I rarely eat the same meals day after day.

   Yes_____   No_____

4. I consistently eat three to five meals per day.

   Yes_____   No_____

5. I rarely skip meals, unless I'm doing intermittent fasting.

   Yes_____   No_____

6. I'm aware of how much protein is recommended for my body size and type, and I usually get the proper amount.

   Yes_____   No_____

7. I make time to eat meals during the day, so I don't play catch-up and snack at night when I'm at home.

   Yes_____   No_____

8. I do NOT rely on soft drinks and high-caffeinated drinks to boost my energy.

   Yes_____   No_____

9. I drink two to three liters of water each day and make sure it's not from the tap unless I live in a place where the water is pristine.

   Yes_____   No_____

10. I can say no to cravings and seconds when I want to.

    Yes_____   No_____

11. Very rarely do I eat greasy or fast foods.

    Yes_____   No_____

12. I take time to reboot my digestive system with digestive enzymes or cleanse my body with fresh juices or fasting periodically.

    Yes_____   No_____

Now, Count your number of "Yes" responses.

Total Score _____

The more YES answers, the higher your standard of excellence for your life vehicle. If you want to improve your health and energy, start with one question and make the change indicated so you have a YES answer.

Coping with Stress and Lifestyle Change

With all the patients and clients I've worked with, and through my own personal experience, I am certain there is a correlation between the way we manage stress and our relationship with food. Some people gorge themselves when stressed, while others skip meals and live on snacks because they're too hassled to shop and prepare proper meals. Chronic stress makes for difficult digestion because the body's adrenaline keeps the sympathetic nervous system activated, which consumes energy necessary for proper digestion to occur. Eating and relaxation need to go together, at least once or twice a day.

If you don't find cooking easy or pleasurable, find a good local restaurant or market that offers healthy take-outs. The food business has come a long way. Today, when you order out, your choices go way beyond pizza and Chinese. Options are abundant, from healthy, fast-food chains to mom-and-pop delis that offer fresh, low-calorie entrees, and now you can get almost anything delivered. So, drop the "I'm too busy to cook" routine and start Googling. The important thing is to always make the healthy decision to eat right, especially when stress and time demands are high. It's never been easier.

So many people start the year with resolutions that include changing their diet and exercise. I like to advise people that the best time to make these resolutions is in the spring or fall: before or after summer vacations and before or after the holiday seasons. If we make eating right a priority in either of these two seasons, then we don't have to gain weight on vacation or lose ten pounds come January and deal with the holiday crash that ensues.

Food, and what we place in our bodies, is one thing we can control. With all the other random and unknowable variables in life, wholesome, nutritious food is something to believe in. The benefits of fueling our bodies with nutritious foods are well researched. While my life has been transformed by giving up "the white stuff," you should test and see if eating less sugar and white flour (and even dairy) make a difference in how you react and process turbulent times. Take steps to master your personal vehicle and treat it with the respect it deserves, and you'll be rewarded with renewed energy, stamina, and confidence.

Chapter 8
Don't Rationalize—Exercise!

*Physical fitness is not only one of the most important keys to a healthy
body, it is the basis of dynamic and creative intellectual activity.*
~John F. Kennedy

Exercise is a living meditation. When you feel sluggish, tired,
or depressed, move the body, and the mind will follow. *Move a
muscle, change a thought* is a fabulous slogan. I don't exercise for my
physique; I exercise for the endorphins that make me feel positive and
upbeat. Along with food, exercise is another variable that you can completely control and is most helpful in times of uncertainty. It's another
example of taking extra care of your body for improved performance and
resiliency in moments of chaos.

In this chapter, we'll explore the various types of exercise to see which
is best tailored to your particular goals. But let's review all the benefits
of exercise to get you excited about what you already do, or what you're
about to add into your self-care regimen.

According to Sara Gottfried, MD, author of *Younger: A Breakthrough
Program to Reset Your Genes, Reverse Aging, and Turn Back the Clock 10
Years*, "Exercise improves sleep, which regulates thousands of genes and
shrinks the white fat that increases your risk of diabetes and heart disease.

Exercise also improves heart function, efficiency, and circulation, lowering the risk of heart disease."

Jillian Michaels, a celebrity-status personal trainer and former host of the popular TV show *The Biggest Loser* was quoted in the *Los Angeles Times* in early 2019, confirming these statistics: "Thirty minutes to an hour of exercise three to four times a week is all you need to increase your vitality and gain a sense of accomplishment."

In the article "Best Anti-Aging Medicine? Exercise" on the website *Everyday Health* (https://www.everydayhealth.com/news/best-anti-aging-medicine-exercise/), Dr. Sanjay Gupta reported that one study found that just fifteen minutes a day of moderate-intensity activity extended people's lives by three years. In a report referenced in the article, Xifeng Wu, MD, professor and chair of The University of Texas department of epidemiology, stated that "exercising at very light levels reduced deaths from any cause by fourteen percent."

Scientific studies show that regular exercise can reduce your physical aging because exercise slows cell aging. Exercise doesn't just make you feel younger—it may actually turn off the aging process in your chromosomes. It has to do with telomeres, the caps at the end of chromosomes that control aging. *If there's a fountain of youth, this is it.* And if there's a fast track to creating calm in chaos, exercise fits the bill.

To further illustrate how exercise keeps us young, in the article "Does Exercise Help Reverse the Effects of Aging?" by Leigh Weingus on the website *MindBodyGreen* (https://www.mindbodygreen.com/0-29265/does-exercise-help-reverse-the-effects-of-aging.html), she states, "Young-looking skin has a lot to do with something called myokines, proteins released by working muscles. The body uses myokines to stay young." So inside and out, exercise benefits our body and helps it to look youthful and function better. Plus, exercise stimulates the hippocampus. Your hippocampus functionality determines your long-term memory— and we all want to have that, far into our old age.

Exercise Hits Home

One of the greatest gifts my mother gave me was the love of exercise. Having had rheumatic fever twice in her childhood, she was bedridden for months at a time. Surviving that, she became a fitness-minded adult. Not only was she athletic through her hobbies of skiing, golfing, tennis, and tai chi, but she also studied karate for fifteen years and became a second-degree black belt at 62 years old. I'm grateful to have had such an example! She stayed active into her 80's with her morning jog, tai chi, tennis, weights, and swimming.

If you have a family history that was lower in exercise discipline or self-care, than you can use that as motivation too. Think of your parents or grandparents, their health issues, and what you want to avoid. Use exercise to counter adverse conditions and break those family ties.

Certain types of movements are designed to promote renewal and inner peace. In general, Western workouts have traditionally been more about tightening and sculpting muscles, while Eastern forms of exercise focus on toning and relaxation. When you carve out time in your schedule for keeping fit, what is your goal? To tighten up or to relax? Or both? Let's dive in a little deeper.

The Best from the West

Different personality and body types tend to benefit from different strategies. I have a girlfriend who releases all her angst after a strenuous Zumba class. She enjoys dance and high-impact movement, so for her, this workout is perfect. Other people prefer weight training, which is the ultimate "tightening" exercise. Actors like Mark Wahlberg and Tom Cruise demonstrate how committed they are to sculpting their bodies. In a TV interview, Mark Wahlberg said he hits the gym at 3:30 a.m. to get his training in before his busy day.

I used to be concerned I'd bulk up if I weight trained, but we all know women who have gorgeous physiques as well. Actresses like Jennifer Lopez and Cameron Diaz kick butt to look fabulous for their high-profile lives and roles. These examples emphasize fitness as a key to successful living. Most high-profile people are pushing the limits not just with their careers but also with their bodies. Singers are another great example of keeping fit for their performance in life. Rolling Stone front man Mick Jagger calls his body *his instrument*, which, by the way he dances, sings, and energizes a stadium, is a pretty accurate assessment. The singer-songwriter P!nk studied and performs on a trapeze as part of her act during concerts.

History of Weight Training

One of the original pioneers of exercise, fitness, and weight training on TV was Jack LaLanne. I have a soft spot for Jack LaLanne because I saw him at a fitness convention in San Diego and he touched my life in one simple hour. He was an advocate for no-sugar living and was so genuine in wanting to lead people to a healthy lifestyle. He told the audience, "Sugar will make you insane."

So here is a little history lesson about what pioneers in fitness or any field go through. When Jack opened his first gym in the 1950's, people gossiped that his ideas were too strange. He wanted to help celebrities and high-level performers, but they scoffed at his ideas of weightlifting and fitness. Instead, he took his gospel of fitness to overweight and troubled youths and began to make a big difference. Suddenly, word got out, and his inspirational message became one of the first exercise programs on television. This was before exercise apps on your phone.

Oprah Winfrey also assisted in the push for healthy living in her high-profile work both with WW (formerly Weight Watchers) and, earlier in her talk show career, when she helped bring "pumping iron" into the limelight when she made the connection with Bob Greene, her personal trainer. Lots of people followed suit and hired personal trainers, and the "boom" is still in full swing. Although weight training doesn't promote relaxation, as do Eastern disciplines, it does provide significant cardiovascular benefits.

Weight Training and Strength Training

As a population, we are concerned with the WIIFM, i.e. what's in it for me. When you choose to do some weight training, you'll strengthen your bones and build muscle too. The latter will speed up your metabolism because muscles burn fat even while you're sleeping. As a bonus, strong muscles and bones reduce the risk of injury and accidents.

In his article "5 Types of Weight Training and their Benefits" on *YogiApproved.com*, Enrico Fioranelli categorized weight training in this way:

1. Total Body Circuit Training

    <u>What it is:</u> This is the traditional boot camp style workout program, with lighter weights in a variety of motions to work out your entire body.

    <u>Who it's good for:</u> Those new to weight training who want to achieve moderate weight loss over an extended period of time.

2. Push-Pull Training

    <u>What it is:</u> Strength training in which you split your routine into different muscle groups and workouts.

    <u>Who it's good for:</u> For moderate to advanced lifters or experienced yogis with good muscle definition.

3. Power Lifting Training

    <u>What it is:</u> Consists of larger movements to incorporate more muscles of your entire body or full-body workout. Examples of these exercises are squats and deadlifts.

    <u>Who it's good for:</u> Advanced strength training if you are looking to become more lean.

4. Explosive Dynamic Training

    <u>What it is:</u> Usually for athletes. Along with an excellent strength and endurance training, these exercises integrate a large car-

diovascular component to get your blood pumping. Examples of these exercises include box jumps, rope pulls, light weight lifting.

Who it's good for: Helps with dynamic weight loss.

5. Muscular Isolation Training

What it is: Working only one-two muscle groups in a day. In this type of program, you will do exercises such as leg extensions, concentration curls, and triceps kickbacks.

Who it's good for: Recommended for advanced lifters or beginners to develop particular muscle groups further. If you're targeting a specific area, i.e. legs or arms to achieve a desired look.

Regardless of your goals, there are weight- and strength-training methods that are perfect for your needs. When you match where you currently are with where you want to be, you can achieve and optimize your results, whether it's sculpted arms or a perfect chaturanga.

Connecting with health-minded people helps us stay committed. When you keep working out and connecting with your friends at the gym, you now have social benefits too. Many people young and old enjoy the camaraderie found at health clubs and exercise classes. It's easier when we work out with others or find a partner to keep us committed. The popular American formula seems to be weight training combined with cardiovascular movement for ultimate health.

Cardiovascular Exercise and Health Benefits:

According to Dr. Johnathan Meyers in his Article "Exercise and Cardiovascular Health" on *ahajournals.org*, the benefits of regular exercise on cardiovascular health include:

- Increase in exercise tolerance
- Reduction in body weight
- Reduction in blood pressure
- Increase in good (HDL) cholesterol

- Reduction in bad (LDL and total) cholesterol
- Boost to immune system
- Regulation of blood sugar level

Let's look at a variety of cardiovascular exercises and how they help you stay healthy.

Brisk walking

Benefits: Brisk walking will help to maintain a healthy weight; prevent or manage various conditions including heart disease, high blood pressure, and type 2 diabetes; improve mood; improve balance and coordination. See MayoClinic.org, "Walking Trims Your Waistline, Improves your Health" (2018)

Running

Benefits: Improves mood, focus, and brain function at any age. Also improves muscles, burns calories, and reduces chances of death. BusinessInsider.com, "8 key ways running can transform your body and brain" (2018) by Kevin Loria.

Swimming

Benefits: Releases body stress; builds endurance, muscle strength and cardiovascular fitness; and helps maintain a healthy weight, heart, and lungs. From betterhealth.vic.gov.au, "Swimming–Health Benefits" by Better Health Channel.

Cycling

Benefits: Provides an aerobic workout; builds muscles; helps with balance, walking, standing, endurance, and stair climbing; increases bone density. From Harvard Health Publishing on health.harvard.edu, "The top 5 benefits of cycling" (August 2016).

Zumba

It is a great fitness program that combines Latin, international, and salsa music with some amazing and fun-filled dance moves. You will find interval training, resistance training, and strength training.

Benefits: Tones your entire body, effectively helps weight loss, great for all ages, reduces stress.

Jazzercise

Famous since the 1970's, this workout offers a great combination of cardio and resistance training. There are over 78,000 Jazzercise instructors today, and weekly Jazzercise classes can be found in almost every country.

Benefits: Reduces the risk of heart disease, gives energy for performance improvement, offers a whole-body workout, helps emotions feel lighter and relaxed.

Ballroom dancing

It is a moderate activity and is popular throughout the world. The only downside with this dance form is that you cannot do it alone. You need a partner for the purpose. Once you have found someone to dance with, you are surely going to have a great experience.

Benefits: Tones muscles, burns calories, boosts confidence, is stress busting and energy boosting, increases bone density, and improves joint flexibility.

Dance Yourself into Fitness

Social benefits arise when you get involved with ballroom dance, Zumba, and Jazzercise. Because of the fun workout that dance provides, attendees often become bonded with instructors and form an exercise tribe. Since Jazzercise paved the way for Tae Bo and Zumba, additional kudos to the founder, Judi Sheppard Missett, and her international organization, Jazzercise.

Wisdom from the East

The popularity of Eastern forms of exercise demonstrates that we Western go-getters also need a change of pace. Yoga, tai chi, chi gong (qigong), and Pilates are available at health clubs throughout the country. Many nationwide chains offer hatha yoga or a Western-like form known as core power yoga. As Americans, we are notorious for taking time-honored practices and modernizing them to better suit our needs. Hence, some forms of yoga are sort of a push-yourself, atta-girl/boy form of the ancient discipline. I prefer the more unadulterated styles of yoga or tai chi. If these forms of exercise have stood the test of time, sign me up. Yoga and tai chi are the world's oldest forms of mental and physical discipline.

Yoga ... Strike a Pose

The Yogic philosophy is one of compassion and connecting with the inner peace that resides in us all. When you do the Yoga postures, you are opening up your body to activate the life force and quiet the mind. Breathing is a key to mental tranquility, and as you do the asanas (Yoga postures), slow deep breathing is part of the "dance."

Ashtanga yoga is about increasing the heat in the body and burning away toxins. The founder of Ashtanga yoga, Sri K. Pattabhi Jois used to say, "Through strenuous poses where the mind has to stay focused, yoga helps to break the negative cycles of the mind that have become chronic thought patterns we fall in love with, even if they're destructive." My teacher, a student of Jois, gave a shorter version *yoga releases the ya yas of the mind.* That's why I enjoyed studio yoga for years, because it was more than an exercise class. Today's technology has brought us apps that are great for travel and time crunches. I hope you get the juicy tidbits I learned in yoga studio classes from the apps because the teacher can lift the students in the class and improve their practice. Hatha yoga is a gentler form of the discipline, popular in the United States, involving more stretching and relaxation techniques. All forms of yoga are designed to bring us into a state of enlightenment, which is why the Yogis have practiced them for centuries. I have to emphasize that the quality of the teacher and your connection with their style is an important factor too. After a class, people should have a glow of *I can't believe how good I feel right now.* Endorphins galore and the relaxing music put us in this state. With the technology at our fingertips, we have an abundance of resources to help us reach this enlightened state, so let's take advantage of them.

The health benefits of yoga include less pain, depression, and anxiety. It provides serenity to better manage stress, improves quality of life in cancer patients, lifts the mood, and helps people reduce their joint or muscular pain.

Tai Chi and Chi Gong

The Chinese have mastered the use of *chi*. Chi is an energy force within us all, and the reservoir of chi is located one inch below the navel and one inch in from the skin. Chinese philosophy teaches that the greater the chi, the healthier the person and the greater their chances for longevity. For thousands of years, the Chinese have performed tai chi with the intention of cultivating the internal life force.

The article "Mind-Body Exercise: Tai Chi and Yoga," on BerkeleyWellness.com, states that the practice of tai chi may provide health benefits such as boosted brain power, less depression and anxiety, better balance and reduced risk of falls, and an overall improved function in people with chronic conditions.

The exercises of tai chi are performed in a standing position and involve very slow specific movements with names like *white crane spreads its wings* and *grasping the bird's tail.* Tai chi is poetry in motion, and just watching a class will relax you. The benefits are exponentially greater for those who participate.

Chi gong is a similar system of activating the life force, but it isn't quite as poetic as the slow chi dance of tai chi. However, chi gong works with meridians of the body. When these energy channels are clear and open, they easily distribute the chi throughout the body. Healthy chi, healthy body. Restricted meridians lead to decreased energy and lower immune function. Chi gong can help people with arm and leg problems.

The Best of All Worlds

According to a National Institutes of Health publication entitled "Health benefits of physical activity: the evidence" (www.ncbi.nlm. nih.gov/pubmed/16534088), exercise has all the following health benefits: lowering blood pressure; reducing the risk of bone and joint diseases, depression, and cardiovascular disease; improving brain function and serotonin levels; and strengthening musculoskeletal fitness which improves posture and metabolic function to offset obesity.

No one else can decide which exercise program is "right" for you. But just as your body benefits from a varied diet, you'll find advantages in trying different types of workouts. If you've never taken a yoga class, you can easily find one at your neighborhood gym or recreation center.

If you find a yoga studio, I suggest you start with a beginner's class. Or you might want to shake up your routine and join the Sierra Club for some hiking. Jumping on a trampoline has become popular, with indoor centers cropping up. If you're near the ocean, riding the waves on a surf or boogie board is a great anecdote to exercise boredom. The most important thing is to keep your body in motion. Whatever you enjoy is what you'll do. Exercise should be a three-letter word because we don't make excuses when we're having f-u-n.

Chapter 9
Alternative Healing Solutions

Albert Einstein called the intuitive or metaphoric mind a sacred gift. He added that the rational mind was a faithful servant. It is paradoxical that in the context of modern life we have begun to worship the servant and defile the divine.

~Bob Samples

Significant research is being done in the field of alternative healing. An office has been established at the National Institute of Health with funding dedicated to determining why and how this phenomenon is taking off. In the U.S. alone, over thirty billion dollars are spent annually on medicinal herbs, vitamins, and nutritional products, and most medical schools now offer classes in alternative healing. Since I've been in this camp for decades, I like to say we are making progress.

I remember when I began studying craniosacral therapy, and John Upledger, DO, FAAO, a physician and passionate craniosacral researcher at the University of Michigan, explained to us, "I attempted to teach this technique to my colleagues. When I showed them the simple manipulations on the cranial bones, they weren't interested. They told me they 'didn't want to touch their patients that much.'" Dr. Upledger was forced to take the technique to hands-on practitioners: physical therapists, chiropractors, dentists, and occupational and massage therapists.

Alternative healing and traditional medicine are still in different camps, but the two are rapidly bridging the gap by sharing their wealth of knowledge. Integrative medicine, which combines the best high-tech Western medicine with alternative approaches, is now being offered at an ever-increasing number of hospitals and medical centers.

I'm heartily recommending alternative techniques for several stress-related conditions. "Stress doesn't only make us feel awful emotionally," says Jay Winner, MD, author of *Take the Stress Out of Your Life* and director of the Stress Management Program for Sansum Clinic in Santa Barbara, California. "It can also exacerbate just about any health condition you can think of." Studies have found many health problems related to stress. "Stress seems to worsen or increase the risk of conditions like obesity, heart disease, Alzheimer's disease, diabetes, depression, gastrointestinal problems, and asthma," according to Dr. Winner's research.

If you don't have a serious health condition now, the techniques introduced here can prevent trouble in the future. If you're flirting with a burnout, been under pressure, or are on the edge of some type of breakdown, these therapies are possible alternatives to pharmaceutical solutions. The idea is to bring the body back naturally to a balanced, healing state.

I've personally experienced each of these modalities and find that, in combination, they help create a calmer presence and greater self-awareness. Several body systems are addressed, and I fully expect that you'll find some better suited to your needs than others. As you work with each technique, you'll become better educated on how to listen to your body through a personally tailored and eclectic approach.

The Benefits of Alternative Healing Methods

1. Your physical awareness becomes heightened.

2. Your emotional, mental, and spiritual issues are addressed simultaneously.

3. Your intuition becomes clearer.

4. Your heightened body awareness makes prevention and self-care easier.

5. Your body is restored to health naturally, without reliance on drugs.

6. You get smarter—even at the cellular level.

7. You experience more compassion and love because it is from this place that healing occurs.

8. You ultimately learn how to activate a healing state on your own, without assistance.

Explore the Healing Recipe for a C.A.L.M. Life.

Each technique is designed to balance the body through touch or movement, or a combination of both.

C is for Chiropractic and Craniosacral Therapy.

Chiropractic Medicine: Chiropractic treatments are now considered pretty much mainstream and are covered by many health plans. Chiropractic care, combined with other alternative therapies, offers a well-balanced approach to health. It addresses the central nervous system by aligning the bones and is based on the theory that the health of the entire body is connected to the condition of the spine. If bones are not aligned properly, the nerve centers that feed various organs and systems (e.g. digestive and respiratory) can't supply the blood and oxygen needed for optimal health. Initial visits can last up to an hour and generally include x-rays. After that, adjustments usually take from ten to thirty minutes.

Indications: Musculoskeletal disorders, including whiplash, lower back pain, sprain or strain, arthritic conditions, sciatica, and neck problems, respond well. Known as organic conditions, headaches, high blood pressure, nervous disorders, and migraines also frequently respond to chiropractic care.

Cost: $50-75 per visit; initial office visit is usually double.

Craniosacral Therapy: This unique therapy addresses the hydraulic system that encloses the brain, spinal cord, cerebrospinal fluid, cranial bones, sacrum, and dura mater membrane. Through gentle manipulations and a light touch, tensions and blocks that create imbalance, dysfunction, and fatigue are released from this central core of the body. Using a process called "unwinding," advanced CST practitioners allow the body to release specific trauma by recreating the body's position when the injury occurred. This can happen spontaneously if the trauma is ready to be corrected and the practitioner follows the craniosacral rhythm. It's no surprise that blocks arising from emotional or physical trauma "hide out" in this central core. When left unaddressed, they become like rocks in a stream, impeding our life force and our full use of sensory faculties. Once released, the body's energy and vitality are restored, and awareness is heightened. This is an effective and spiritual approach to healing the body. Treatments take from one to two hours.

Indications: Several conditions can benefit from CST: headaches, nervous problems, TMJ, back pain, ear and eye disorders, depression, learning disabilities, chronic fatigue syndrome, and hyperactivity.

Cost: $85- $150 per hour

A is for Acupuncture and the Alexander Technique.

Acupuncture: This well-known Eastern technique uses needles to open the meridians of the body. These meridians are energy channels that allow the life force called "chi" to activate and energize us. Vital people have an abundance of this life force pulsing throughout their system. Acupuncturists make diagnoses by listening to the pulses in the wrists, noting the color of the tongue, and assessing symptoms. They then determine which points they will stimulate with extremely thin (almost hair-like) acupuncture needles. (Those who normally turn pale at the sight of a syringe needn't worry—this is *not* like getting an injection.) Sometimes a small battery-powered electrical device is used to provide more stimulation to open blocked energy centers. Another enhancement is moxibustion, a cigar-shaped stick made of Chinese mugwort. Once ignited, this stick acts as a heat source to stimulate the needles activating the chi at various points.

Indications: Pain, organ imbalances, headaches, allergies, asthma, back problems, stress, nervous conditions, insomnia, impotence, frozen shoulder, and joint problems. Treatments usually take thirty to sixty minutes and are both relaxing and revitalizing.

Cost: $65-$125 per treatment

Alexander Technique: F. Matthias Alexander was an aspiring actor with a promising career when he developed vocal difficulties. His doctors didn't have a solution, so he began observing his neck and head in the mirror while speaking. He concluded that faulty postural habits were creating his vocal dysfunction. After healing his voice, he helped others to alter incorrect or inefficient physical habits that cause stress and fatigue.

Through a series of lessons to improve one's awareness of movement patterns, this technique addresses the unconscious misuse of the body in performing everyday tasks. This technique recognizes the maintenance of the neck muscles and position of the head as primary requirements for efficient use of the body. Relaxation techniques and simple exercises to retrain the muscles are used to improve posture.

Indications: Popular among professional athletes, musicians, dancers, and actors, this technique also serves those with various types of ongoing pain.

Cost: $80-$125 per session, usually one hour. Group classes are less expensive.

L is for Lomilomi Massage and Lymph Drainage Therapy.

Lomilomi Massage: "Auntie" Margaret Machado learned this technique from those who attended to Hawaiian royalty, and she shared it with the rest of the healing world. A relaxing and invigorating form of Hawaiian massage, steeped in ancient tradition, it breaks up muscle spasms with a series of movements of the hands, forearms, and elbows. The strokes are done with the hands and forearms and are often long and sweeping, much like long, rolling waves traveling along the body.

In an article on MassageMagazine.com titled "Lomilomi Massage: The Art of Hawaiian Sacred Healing" by Gloria Coppola, LMT (https://www.massagemag.com/lomilomi-hawaiian-massage-87100/), she explains:

> The foundation of lomilomi in many lineages includes the practice of a martial art, *lua*, which builds strength, focus, endurance and discipline. … Lomilomi also includes range-of-motion work, deep-tissue techniques and, most importantly, the full presence of loving touch. Every cell is blessed to create balance (*lokahi*). The nervous system is encouraged to slow down, thereby creating the space for techniques to be received rather than pushing through a blockage in the muscle tissue. Creating movement in the spine is a primary focus of lomilomi. One might even experience unwinding similar to that which occurs in myofascial release.

The overall effect is very nurturing, touching the heart through the practitioner's hands. Sessions incorporate physical and spiritual aspects of healing, allowing the body to release stress and toxins.

Indications: Beneficial for musculoskeletal disorders, pregnancy, muscle tension, and stress relief. This technique's nurturing quality helps heal emotional loss and grief.

Cost: $75-$155 per hour. 75- to 90-minute sessions are recommended.

Lymph Drainage Therapy: You might call the lymph system the body's "garbage disposal." This wonder fluid runs through the body, wherever there is blood. Responsible for detoxification of the tissues, it is also the pathway of cellular immunity for B-cells and T-cells. Whether we're fighting cancer or the common cold, it is the lymph system's effectiveness that bolsters immunity and fights infection. This method, developed by Bruno Chikly, MD, effectively stimulates the lymphatic flow, opening up the lymph system of those with chronic edema and autoimmune diseases. When lymph isn't moving efficiently, our body becomes toxic and can produce mental, physical, and emotional imbalances. In an LDT session, selected points are stimulated, moving stagnant lymph and inflation by increasing lymph circulation through the body. One should drink plenty of water before and after a session to maximize the cleansing effect. Sessions are relaxing and regenerating and stimulate the parasympathetic function.

Indications: Inflammatory disorders such as bronchitis, sinusitis, arthritis, acne, eczema, and chronic fatigue syndrome; it also helps depression and attention-deficit/hyperactivity disorder.

Cost: $90-150 per session

For more information on Lymph Drainage Therapy, you can order Dr. Chikly's book, *Silent Waves: Theory and Practice of Lymph Drainage Therapy*, currently in its third edition. It can be purchased through Amazon or IAHE, (800) 233-5880.

M is for Acupressure and Swedish Massage

All massage stimulates the parasympathetic function of the body. Here are some of the benefits listed in Dr. Chikly's book regarding parasympathetic function. It is generally most active during sleep and deep relaxation states, and it conserves and helps restore body energy, regenerating injured tissues.

Benefits:

1) Stimulates immune functions
2) Decreases heart rate
3) Decreases respiratory rate
4) Decreases blood pressure
5) Increases blood flow to the skin
6) Increases blood sugar level
7) Increases gastrointestinal motility and kidney function
8) Increases digestive gland function
9) Increases bronchial gland function
10) Increases salivary gland function

Acupressure Massage: This treatment uses the same principle of activating energy centers and meridian points as acupuncture, but stimulation occurs through touch rather than piercing of the skin. (This is great for those who get white knuckles even at the *thought* of a needle!)

Muscular tension accumulates around acupressure points, which causes muscle groups to contract and block the flow of vital life force throughout the body.

Indications: Menstrual problems, migraine headaches, insomnia, digestive disorders, backaches, and muscular pain are some of the maladies that respond well to this treatment.

Cost: $75-$150 per hour session

Swedish Massage: One of the most popular massage techniques, commonly offered in health clubs and spas. It includes a variety of strokes—kneading, shaking, light percussion, and cross-friction—addressing the entire body. It is designed to wake up or energize the body through increased circulation. Benefits include relief for sore muscles, improved circulation, reduced swelling, and overall relaxation. A bonus is a mood lift because Swedish massage stimulates endorphins.

Indications: Fatigue, depression, sore muscles, pregnancy, headaches, stiff necks, back and shoulder pain, fluid retention, and insomnia.

<u>Cost</u>: $50-$125 per hour

(Experience counts here. Most massage therapists start with Swedish and then add other techniques as they gain experience.)

The Importance of Energy Alignment

When we visit a practitioner, it's vital that we feel relaxed in his or her presence. Even if someone comes highly recommended, if you don't feel completely comfortable, then you need to find another source. Your well-being should be a practitioner's top priority, and their presence should be comforting and confident as they work to open your blocks and energy imbalances. Once that is established, fantastic results can occur.

When we feel out of balance, we're at a disadvantage, because in times of vulnerability we tend to lose our normal sense of discernment and clarity. During times of chaos, we can grant health practitioners too much power, which can be dangerous if we happen across someone unscrupulous. Except in a medical emergency, we should never turn our entire well-being over to the care of someone else. It is not the job of any one doctor or health-care practitioner to restore and heal us. *That is our job.* We must select our experts carefully and take responsibility for our choice of treatments.

If someone recommends a treatment that strikes us as absurd—it probably is. And try to avoid prescriptions that create more toxins in the body and an even greater need for alternative healing. In addition to good common sense, here are a few guidelines.

Nine Things to Look for in an Alternative Healing Practitioner

1. Positive, uplifting energy and presence
2. Understanding, easy to relate to
3. Good communicator
4. Provides professional materials and literature

5. Provides a pleasant, calming environment
6. Focuses on you and your specific needs
7. Considerate of your time
8. May offer—but doesn't push—additional products or services
9. Willing to accommodate you in a crisis

(If fees are higher than average, services should be exceptional and customized. Lower-than-average fees may reflect a sacrifice in one or more of the areas listed above. Resort spas charge premium rates but also hire exceptional therapists!)

Having been both a patient and a practitioner for years, I've heard a lot of stories and have a few of my own. Here are a couple of cautionary tales to assist you in making wise choices.

The Pushy Practitioner

My favorite practitioner owned a health center that was thirty-plus minutes away. With my busy schedule, I rationalized I didn't need to do the one-hour drive to go to someone I completely connected with. So, I decided to work with a health center that was closer to my home, and I found someone local. After my first session, this new practitioner tried to convince me I needed to come back in one day. Wow, here I am a health professional getting someone trying to push me into extra services. I might have left then, but I didn't. The next thing I know, she has a new line of supplements and starts pushing them on me. It's an interesting paradigm because the day I was the most vulnerable is the day she succeeded in selling me. When we are looking for healing, we are in a vulnerable state vs. a strong one. It was clear she wanted me as a client for purposes that served her more than me.

It's tricky when we try to save time and/or money, and these types of practitioners can take advantage. That is the reason I share this experience. I also learned that we all make mistakes at times on who we spend our dollars with. Please don't allow a bad experience to stop you from getting your needs met. Move on and believe you will find the right one. This same scenario can happen with traditional medical professionals, so be aware. Sometimes people can sense when they can take advantage, like in this next story.

Trust Your Instincts, Not a Doctor's Ego

In my earlier years of studying Buddhism for a short time, I came home from a week-long spiritual retreat in England. The lessons I learned that summer were unexpected, and my body felt out of sorts. I felt so vulnerable that I sought out someone new to help me. My first choice was a chiropractor that was also an acupuncturist. On my initial visit, he seemed extremely confident and boasted about the uniqueness of his method. He claimed he could cure the pain in my neck, still stressed from earlier whiplash injuries. He convinced me that I needed adjustments *twice a week*. This was about six sessions more per month than I'd had in the past. But this man was so convincing that I followed his advice—in spite of nagging doubts.

Within a short time, I experienced the worst pain I'd ever known: migraine-like headaches, lower back pain, and an overall sense of disorientation. Finally, I realized that this practitioner was more interested in advancing his business (and his bank account) than in serving my needs.

Affording Services on a Tight Budget

The field of alternative health is one where you can find sliding-scale fees and community center services that are significantly cheaper. Acupuncture clinics have community days one or two times a month. You don't get a private room, but you get your treatment at a reduced cost. Massage schools offer student massages at half price. Also, if you have a disease, like breast cancer, several spas nationwide offer their facilities and talent at no charge one night a month. You can get the health benefits you need within your circumstances; just be determined. If you have financial stress, you have additional stress.

There are still those who think anything outside the realm of traditional medicine is primitive or downright flaky. The truth is, we need both allopathic medical doctors and alternative health practitioners to maintain a healthy mind and body. I certainly don't recommend that anyone stop seeing their medical doctor. I'm just suggesting that if you aren't getting the results you want, and medical tests aren't shedding enough light on your condition, it might be time to try the alternative approach. With all the chaos going on in this world today, maybe this book will help you take a leap, so you can open your mind, read, learn, and, when you're ready, enjoy health maintenance services. You deserve to feel connected and whole and to enjoy every day of your life to the fullest.

Chapter 10
Spiritual Healing Solutions and Prayer Power

One moon dispels the darkness of the heavens.
Similarly, one soul who is trained to know God, a soul in whom
there is true devotion and sincere seeking and intensity, will dispel
the spiritual darkness of others wherever he will go.
~Paramahansa Yogananda

As I mentioned in the previous chapter, alternative healing opens us up to greater awareness, intuition, and calming energy. For many, it's a welcome relief to tune in to life at a deeper level. However, the more open and compassionate you become, the more protection and self-assessment skills you need to maintain this inner peace.

As open and peaceful vessels of light in a sometimes dark and chaotic world, we may find ourselves feeling vulnerable and in need of protection. When we're standing up to serve humanity's highest good, we shouldn't have to live in a state of worry. Protection, in the sense I'm using it here, is an ancient wisdom, and it has nothing to do with a bodyguard.

Talismans

When warriors of old went into battle, they often carried a talisman for protection. A Saint Christopher medal for Catholics is another example, and some Native Americans wear beautiful stones to complement various medicines. Some people like scriptures, e.g. "Guard your heart above all else, for it determines the course of your life." Prov. 4:23.

One of my clients used to buy a lot of Native American jewelry, looking for just the right piece. After years of searching, she finally came across a grizzly claw fashioned to wear as a pendant. Since she had a strong belief in Native American animal medicines, she felt a great sense of protection in this magical, ornament-like talisman.

While taking a break from writing and editing this book, I went to an art center in Palm Springs. I enjoyed walking the whole gallery. As I was getting ready to leave, an artist showed up with pendants hand-carved out of buffalo bone. There were all different styles, but the one I kept trying on depicted a bear surrounding a sage medicine woman. Oh, these pieces weren't run-of-the-mill, factory-produced products. You could feel the power and spirituality that had been infused in each pendant by a woman who was both artist and medicine woman. I purchased this Native American beaded talisman pendant named Bear Woman, and it gave me everything I needed to finish writing and editing this book.

Be it prayer beads or a family heirloom necklace, special ring, smooth crystal, lucky coin, mass card, note, or love letter, a personal talisman can help you feel grounded and calm around chaotic people and situations. Let's face it, we like to have protection, and we feel helped by certain items that we sense give us a little magical support. It can be clothing articles too! So, dear ones, if you are feeling vulnerable and not as strong as you'd like, maybe there is a talisman you need to seek out. Check out *www.riseabovethechaos.com* for healing products and resources to help you.

The Importance of the Biofield

The energetic nature of our being and the challenging world in which we live mean that constant daily attention needs to be paid to the energies that we are. Caring for our energetic self is as much a vital aspect of daily self-care as cleaning our teeth, especially if we are striving for vibrant health.

In 1994, the National Institute of Health chose the term "biofield" to describe the field of energy and information that surrounds and inter-penetrates the human body. The biofield is recognized as being composed of veritable (electromagnetic) and putative (subtle) energies. The biofield conveys information for organizing the human body and is thought to regulate the biochemistry and physiology.

Whenever we experience any type of trauma, it affects our biof-ield; this can be seen by gifted energy healers. The trauma may appear in the biofield as an area of density, or an area of fragmentation. If the areas of the biofield holding the effects of the trauma are not addressed, that is likely to adversely affect our physical, emotional, or mental health.

There are many energy medicine approaches, like those discussed in Chapter 9: Alternative Healing Solutions, that can be incorporated into your life-balance protocols in order to address this most fundamental, yet often omitted, spiritual and energetic component to wellness.

At some of the premier health shows where I speak and exhibit, I have connected with Barbara Evans, the gifted artist, minister, and healer who created beautiful Healing Chakra Discs. I have been so impressed with her work. One day, her company sent out an announce-ment that she had a new product for healing the biofield, called Per-sonal Empowerment Discs.

I immediately purchased her Personal Empowerment Discs over the internet, sight unseen. Having met her several times, I knew instinc-tively I needed them. Although I attempted to resist buying the full set,

I eventually realized I needed all of them. Each one represents a different property: Healing, Abundance, Wisdom, Joy, New Dreams, Love.

Just making the purchase made me feel so excited, like I had just purchased something very important. Once they arrived, I immediately set them up by the Creative Life Solutions sign in my office. Within a month, I was taking all kinds of empowered steps: hiring a New York editor, buying the car of my dreams, creating "Rise Above the Chaos" videos for YouTube, and planning a book tour. I was rapidly achieving several goals I'd been longing for.

The Personal Empowerment Discs simply need to be within our energy field for the beneficial energetic interaction to begin. If you meditate, you can hold them and sense the beneficial energies in the palm of your hand. The discs are in a form that is very attractive and easy to use, as they help to clear, heal, strengthen, and maintain the energetic self.

Do You Have an Altar in Your Home?

Do you ever feel bombarded by technology? Plasma screens here, computers there, routers, cell phones, microwaves, etc. There is a lot going on in our Wi-Fi world and our homes aren't immune to it, unless we live off the grid.

I've always had a "special place" in all my homes. I like to think of it as an altar, but I'm not talking about the Catholic church with deities. If you are looking to improve the biofield in your dwelling and rise above the chaos, perhaps this is a tool that will help you. Find a place you look at regularly and set a specific intention that the objects you place there are to protect and inspire you in special ways. What about photos of a loved one who you feel watches over you?

People who are attracted to crystals and minerals might place these objects at their home altar to protect their environment. Minerals that are strengthening and uplifting include amethyst, chrysocolla, citrine, fluorite, jade, labradorite, and tourmaline.

Tools for a Lifted Spirit and Life

It is lovely to have sacred objects and photos, but let's go a bit deeper in fortifying ourselves when we need to really rise above things that are pushing us down.

I frequently ask God for protection when I need to complete projects or attend events where I know my energy will be on full-steam-ahead and potentially challenged. Again, in working with cancer patients, I think you can gather I've had to learn a few tricks over the years. How do we access this protection?

In some of my Day of Healing seminars, I offer a guided meditation where I ask people to call up their special protection, and afterward I invite participants to share their experience. Some people see glorious visualizations that they continue to call upon. One person saw himself sheltered by a pair of cupped hands that emitted a swirl of energy. Another envisioned a translucent bubble that was flexible and iridescent, reflecting a rainbow of colors. This bubble surrounded her and pushed all negative energy away. Another woman pictured herself enveloped in a flame of red, gold, and white. Still others saw a purple or violet flame and felt a crackling presence that evaporated anything that drew near.

The Gift of Clairvoyance

The gift of inner sight is called clairvoyance, and those who see Angels and energy fields called "auras" have this special talent. One of the world's best-known clairvoyants was an American named Edgar Cayce. When people came to him seeking relief from illness, he could go into a trance and locate the origin of the disease. He is said to have cured people whom doctors had failed. Word of his gift spread, and he eventually had to get an unlisted number because people were constantly calling him. If strangers came to him in anger, he would see their rage before they approached, and he requested that they return when their emotions were under control. This is the way he protected himself.

I learned a lot about dealing with those in chaos while working in a hospital setting where you can't tell people to go away. Instead, you cultivate the skills to protect yourself, and you dodge the negative emotions of people who are enveloped in depression, self-pity, anxiety, anger, and entitlement.

Spiritual Seeker

I don't think I consciously chose to work with those who are suffering, but it's obvious to me now that my life was preparing me for this. I was always seeking spiritual teachers and methods. This helped me cope with not only my own family, but later with all the families I would work with as a patient advocate.

I've been blessed to study with mystics and those who have developed these spiritual gifts since I was in my 20's, from the teaching of Flower Newhouse, the founder of The Christward Ministry and author of a multitude of books on the Angel Kingdom, to Ann Meyer Makeever, the founder of the Teaching of the Inner Christ, teaching us to access that Christ Vibration and offer it to the world to help those in need, to by far my personal favorite, my "spiritual mother," Reverend Dr. Judith Larkin Reno, founder of Gateway University and the innovator of the God Ladder, which explained stages of spiritual initiation.

All of these sacred churches and teachers opened up my own gifts to serve humanity. Intuition and clairvoyance can come from inner sight rather than external vision and are greatly enhanced with regular prayer and meditation practices. Some people call those who have these skills prophets, but really, we all can access these higher octaves if we train and develop ourselves. It takes time and work, but if you want to rise above *any* chaos, this is where I'd start.

My first choice is prayer, the greatest protector of all for those who are able to humble themselves and ask for strength and fortification. Second, we can take some quiet time in the morning or evening to meditate. In this "listening" place, we can ask how we can be shielded from chaos and be strengthened so we feel protection in ourselves. Third, we can simply ask. "Seek and ye shall find." Fourth, we can find a way to forgiveness and make it a daily practice.

Prayer Power

If you don't think prayer can provide peace, think for a moment about the late Mother Teresa. If you don't believe prayer gives you strength to overcome adversity, remember Rose Kennedy, the matriarch who lost a daughter and three sons in her lifetime, including the thirty-fifth president of the United States, John F. Kennedy. And if you don't think prayer gives you wisdom, consider the Dalai Lama.

Even those who pray frequently sometimes forget to pray in moments of chaos. Yet it is an effective way to the "release that leads to peace" in critical moments, especially if you remember to pray before taking the next indicated step. For the last decade, I've relied on a series of prayers to change my psyche about who I am and what I deserve.

One of my favorite classic movie lines comes from the film *Shadowlands* about the life of C.S. Lewis, portrayed by Anthony Hopkins. After a long life as a bachelor, C.S. Lewis finally falls in love and marries. Some time later his wife is diagnosed with cancer. As he leaves a chapel after hearing her prognosis, one of his colleagues offers condolences, and Lewis replies, "All I can do is pray. I don't pray to change God; I pray to change me for God."

My purpose here is not to tell you how to pray, but rather to urge you to pray. I'm going to share some of my personal prayers that I have used to change me for God, and you can use them, if you wish, as a guide for your own prayer work. If, in the past, you haven't found prayer fulfilling, I recommend that you give prayer another chance until you find a method that works for you.

It's always good to go before the Creator with your own words and thoughts. After all, we are created in the Creator's image. Throughout the ages, Christian mystics and devoted spiritualists have given us beautiful words of inspiration. But sometimes we have to find our own.

The shortest prayer I've ever prayed was during my father's five weeks as a quadriplegic. I was so emotionally drained after his accident that all I could say was: *God help me!* But it worked. Soon after, a dear friend sent me a beautiful cassette and video titled *In Search of Angels,* and its music fortified and comforted me during that critical time.

Sometimes we need special prayers for specific situations. Before I board an airplane, I always say a Christian Science prayer that I learned from my great grandmother: *Around, beneath, and above are the everlasting arms of love.* When I'm running late and in need of a parking space, I sometimes say, *Love makes radiant room.* And the well-known Serenity Prayer is a longtime favorite; I often turn to it when my mind is racing with unresolved issues in the middle of the night or day: *God grant me the serenity to accept the things I cannot change, the courage to change the things I can, and the wisdom to know the difference.*

My "quick" version of the Prayer of St. Francis almost always creates a positive difference in my attitude:

> Make me an instrument of thy peace
> That where there is hatred I may bring love,
> Darkness…Light
> Discord…Harmony.

The complete prayer is a joy to read:

> Lord, make me an instrument of thy peace.
> Where there is hatred, let me bring love.
> Where there is offense, let me bring pardon.
> Where there is discord, let me bring union.

Where there is error, let me bring truth.

Where there is doubt, let me bring faith.

Where there is darkness, let me bring your light.

Where there is sadness, let me bring joy.

O Master, let me not so much seek to be consoled

As to console,

To be understood as to understand,

To be loved as to love,

For it is in giving that one receives,

It is in self-forgetting that one finds,

It is in pardoning that one is pardoned,

It is in dying

That one is raised to eternal life.

Customize Your Prayer Treatments

Writing my own prayer treatments has been paramount in putting my consciousness before God for transforming. For years I have used the formula taught by Ernest Holmes and the teachings of Religious Science to prepare my mind for change. When I healed my cancer in 2003, I believe this was where my mental work prepared me to help others. The benefit of these Spiritual Mind Treatments is that my mind gets aligned with higher wisdom and purpose. If you are seeking to know more about Ernest Holmes, the website is www.csl.org; his centers are nationwide.

Here are the steps and a sample of one of my prayers:

1. Seek
2. Align
3. Claim
4. Accept
5. Express Gratitude

Prayer for the Power of the Spoken Word

Seek

I begin my prayer seeking higher wisdom and guidance. I declare the characteristics of that higher wisdom and power, and in so doing, I am lifted beyond my problems.

"I recognize God as the source that operates all life. Universal unity, creator, orchestrator, and designer of all life; all-encompassing love, ever-present clarity, guidance, and wisdom are the essence of God."

Align

I now declare the characteristics of that higher wisdom and power within me and expressed in my life. From this vantage point, the words I speak will have affirming power. All words have power, but these words have a strong and special intent.

"I am the source that operates all life. I am universal unity, creator orchestrator, and designer of all life. All-encompassing love is the essence of me, ever-present clarity, guidance, and wisdom are the essence of me."

Claim

I now state the solution, ideal, or goal I wish to attain. As I state my desire, I add the clause "or better" at the end. This is important because from my human perspective, I cannot see the big picture and don't always know what is best. (Surprise!)

"I claim that I now express the power of my spoken and written words, as a professional speaker and writer. Audiences are lifted to clarity, resiliency, and purposeful power. Well-matched clients and opportunities are continuously flowing into my business, allowing me to act as a people developer and a resource to help people rise above the chaos and restore the infrastructure of people's lives now, or better."

Accept

This is where I change me—my mind. I state words that release any limitations or blocks in me, then I claim that I am ready to accept and able to receive the outcome I'm praying for. This should be the longest part of the prayer because the purpose is to develop conviction that every possible obstacle is removed and resolved, to build confidence that this outcome—or an even better one—is certain to occur.

"I release all my fears of deficiency. I know the power of my spoken word is divinely directed and revealing. I consciously select the words I speak and the thoughts I send out into the biofield, knowing that how I perceive life is what I experience. I perceive only the best in myself and others; therefore, my life is a continual expansion, refinement, and conduit for great good. I align my consciousness with God's light and allow any self-doubt to be cleared from me and lifted into the light. I know that I am an agent of change, privileged to assist in carrying out God's plan. I release all false notions that I'm not enough to carry the spoken and written word to others. I embrace all my skills and field-tested self-esteem. I embrace the fact that I chose to be an instrument for good. I release the false idea that being a powerful teacher is too demanding. I realize God is power. I allow this power to live through me now and protect me at all times. I release all false beliefs that I'm too weak, inconsistent, or undisciplined to manifest a successful speaking, coaching, and publishing career. Profound work is being accomplished in my life and business now, or better. I align my life with God's will in an orderly fashion. The voice of God is the voice in me. God is the source of my power and my message. I know that I am God's trusted instrument and I focus on aligning my life with Universal Good. I work consistently to prepare myself, and to demonstrate healing, health, and success in my life and in the lives of the people I work for, write for, work with, love, and cherish."

Express Gratitude

Here I express my gratitude for the results I am praying for. I thank my higher power as if I had already received the desired outcome.

"Thank you, wonderful God, for fulfilling my life dream, by guiding every step of my speaking journey as a trusted orator, coach, business woman, and consummate communicator."

Use these prayers to guide and inspire you. Each of us prays in our own unique manner, and it is my hope that each of you will find your own special way of utilizing this remarkable and often miraculous power.

Prayer Partners

Sometimes it helps to have a prayer partner. It makes us stay true to the course of consistent prayer. We have someone with whom we can share the realizations and manifestations. My joyous prayer partner for several years would teach me little tricks like *let's pray for forty days*. She was well-versed in the Bible and believed this was significant. She also gave me this gem: a prayer for guidance. I feel such a release as I pray this before I go out into the day. It continues to bring me great results. I hope it does the same for you!

Guidance Prayer

Show me where to go
Show me who to meet
Give me the words to say
And Lord keep me out of your way
Show me who I can help today

New Year's Blessing by Rev. Dr. Judith Larkin Reno

Going forward may Angels hold you in their embrace
And fill you with their grace

May you rivet your focus on God, so you always walk with the
wise and strong
May the Holy Spirit emblazon and empower you
Let tender mercies prevail in your year ahead and always
Even as the hand of God holds the Earth in space
May you realize that you are personally supported by that same
divine power
And love and infinite supply

Chapter 11
Restore, Relax, Renew

The soul gives us resilience—an essential quality since we constantly have to rebound from hardship.
~Wynton Marsalis

This chapter spotlights my ten favorite techniques to restore, relax, and renew your body and soul. Spiritual self-care is an essential tool in your arsenal to fight off the ill effects of toxic people and our turbulent times. Today's fast-paced chaos causes us to become stressed, alienated from our true selves, and eventually jaded. And when we're jaded, we lose touch with our body and soul. We forget that we're made of stardust and connected to everything in the Universe. We lose sight of what feeds our soul. We sleepwalk through life, detached from our true selves and higher purpose.

To get back to our natural state of balance and alignment with our higher power, we must turn to both alternative *and* spiritual healing. Alternative healing helps update our hard drive so we can keep producing as a human-*doing*. Spiritual healing frees up the heaviness in our soul. When we practice specific self-care solutions, we keep our life in balance by connecting to our human-*being*.

I hope this chapter will encourage you to become more intimately in touch with your breathing and to harness the power of community and loving and supportive friends. It's time to get grounded with the Earth and your tribe. It's time to find peace in your body. It's in these still moments where you will find inner strength and be blessed with grace.

Running on Empty

There is a series of health shows I do annually over back-to-back weekends that take all of my emotional, spiritual, and physical strength. I'm focused, present, and engaged, and with all that is involved, it's a big undertaking. I can be certain I'll need to restore myself once these shows are completed.

This past year it was the same routine, and as I finished my last presentation, I felt relieved, but not spent. I didn't realize I had been running on pure adrenaline and not listening to my body. When the fatigue and crash undeniably set in, I knew it was time for self-care.

I had a stack of client emails to answer, associates in my office who needed my time, and a husband and family who were rightly looking for attention. In the past, I might have jumped from the stage lights right back into the daily drama of work and family life balance. But I know now that without my brain, body, and spirit intact, I'm no help to anyone. This has been a hard lesson to learn: to recognize that self-care is not *selfish* but *selfless*. You can't help others or do your best work if you're disjointed, exhausted, and spent.

So, I looked to restore, relax, and renew. I started my self-care plan with a couple of days off, a longer-than-normal massage, and a chiropractic adjustment. Assuming I'd be fresh and fine, I was surprised when I wasn't. So, I went down my C.A.L.M. list (see Chapter 9) and decided to get some acupuncture. Sure enough, the restore was my chiropractic adjustment, relax was the massage, and renew was acupuncture.

It was during my treatment when the acupuncturist stated, "Oh, I can tell you've been working hard; it's time to reset yourself." So, when we do *all of the above*, we reset ourselves. That is what this entire book is designed to do.

Reset is One Letter from Rest

Too many of us push self-care to the bottom of our to-do list, if it's even on it at all. All too often, we place the health and emotional needs of others before ourselves. There are times when this is necessary, but if you don't eventually get back in balance, there is a price to pay. Hitting the reset button should be celebrated as a sacred act of love. Right now, we put up too many obstacles before finding the time or money to hit the reset button appropriately. Whether you're a stay-at-home dad or a financial executive, we all face this dilemma. The more responsibility you have in life, the more often you need to get back on track.

I had the privilege of touring a submarine that had been used in World War II to invade the Japanese waters. (The museum at Pearl Harbor is must-see for those who visit Hawaii.) This was the lead submarine that the others on the mission followed. In touring the ship, I marveled at how the quarters were so confined; these men had barely any privacy to eat, sleep, or dwell on their own. As crowded and regimented as this existence was, the tour passed this room that looked like a decent hotel room with a private entrance, bed, desk, and mirror.

Then the tour guide explained those were the Captain's quarters, which are spacious and separated from the crew, because he had to make decisions that involved the lives of all the men onboard the submarine and the six others that followed them. That message and image have stayed with me as my favorite example of why highly stressful jobs require quiet time for restoration.

From Robotic to Authentic

One of my mentors in the speaking business regales audiences with tales of her fast-track days. During her early years, she worked incredibly hard, scheduling every minute for optimal productivity. She admits that after a few years at breakneck speed, she began to feel like a robot. Reading through her daily agenda of sales calls, speaking engagements, and staff meetings, she jokes that she even used to schedule in time for lovemaking with her husband.

She would recite in a robotic voice: "10:00-10:20 p.m.—Make love with Larry. Oops! He's late. Gotta start without him!" Audiences always roar with laughter when she tells this story. Can't we all relate?

But my friend touches a nerve in almost everyone because she's kidding on the square. Most of us know at some level that there's certainly a joie de vivre that gets lost in the shuffle when we over-schedule ourselves. But pressures mount, and we do what we feel we have to do. When we finally take a breather from the robot track and take time to restore ourselves, we become more authentic. By allowing time for human-*being*, without human-*doing*, we can rediscover our inner rhythms of productivity and creativity and our instincts about what's right for *us*.

I've noticed consistently in my life that I often will think that the one more thing I just can't fit in is something that's essential for *me*. I can't squeeze in that yoga class or going to a wellness event. When I'm in a robotic mode, I often forget to listen to my heart. At the end of a yoga class recently, the instructor prompted us, saying, "Take your right hand put it over your heart. Your right hand represents your mind. Now take your left hand and place it over your right hand and heart. Your left hand represents your heart." Then with both hands touching our heart, she said, *"Remember to use both your mind and your heart equally as you make your decisions and choices in life."*

Ten Steps to Restore, Relax, Renew

Here are ten ways you can use your physical senses to nurture your body, mind, and soul, and reset to live your life's highest purpose.

1. Laughter Power

It's obvious, right? To rise above the chaos, you have to lighten up. Why not laugh about it too? Life can be beautifully absurd. If you can find a bit of lightness in even the darkest of times, laughter can illuminate the way. And don't forget that flood of endorphins released with those belly laughs that help reset the brain.

One of my earliest California memories was being the catering director at San Diego State University and securing a contract for the summer concerts. Well, the surprise was that one of the performances wasn't a musician, but a comedian: Robin Williams. God, rest his soul. I know he had bumps to overcome during his life, but his talent was astonishing to see up close. This guy was full-on laughter power. He loved to laugh, and he loved, even more, to make you laugh. His fellow comedians could barely hold on, as watching him was everyone's delight.

You can't be depressed when you're laughing. You can't worry about relationships, money, or health when you're laughing. That's why I'm so inspired by the work of Dr. Madan Kataria, a medical doctor from India who created the Laughter Yoga University and practice that has spread across one hundred countries. Dr. Kataria took the simple concept that the brain cannot tell the difference between fake and real laughter and developed a playful practice of breathing exercises and games to release those feel-good hormones.

"The concept of Laughter Yoga is based on a scientific fact that the body cannot differentiate between fake and real laughter. One gets the same physiological and psychological benefits. Clinical research conducted at Bangalore, India, and in the United States has proved that laughter lowers the level of stress hormones (epinephrine, cortisol, etc.) in the blood." (https://laughteryoga.org/)

Laughter is indeed powerful medicine. Whether it's a laughing yoga class, a comedy show, or YouTube pet videos, find what tickles your funny bone and see how it keeps you moving forward. And the next time people are expecting you to get stressed or upset, try laughing. You'll feel better and amaze your audience.

2. Water Power.

Water rules our planet. Our bodies are seventy-six percent water. Without it, we quickly die. Dr. F. Batmanghelidj's book, *Your Body's Many Cries for Water*, documents an array of afflictions including back problems, arthritis, heart disease, and hormone imbalances that can be reversed by keeping the body properly hydrated. The importance of drinking water (roughly two quarts a day) cannot be stressed enough. Water washes and nourishes our bodies from the inside out. Try drinking an extra quart of water once a week and see if you notice the difference.

Dehydration will slow your metabolism and can cause fatigue and even depression. People sometimes mistake the thirst mechanism for hunger. The next time you're hungry, try drinking a sixteen-ounce glass of water. This has been a dieter's secret for years: The more water you drink, the less food you'll crave. And don't worry about water reten-tion. The body hoards water when we get *too little* and discards it when it gets enough.

Please don't think other liquids will replace the need for water. Caf-feine and alcohol have a mild diuretic effect. So, if you indulge, become a two-fisted drinker: Down some extra water for each glass of wine or cup of coffee. (Note: If your water intake is currently low, it's best to increase it gradually, adding a glass or two a day until you reach eight.)

What do swimming pools, Jacuzzis, oceans, rivers, and streams all have in common? These various sources of water can clear and restore the body. Even if we don't immerse ourselves in water, we feel better just being in the presence of a lovely river, lake, or stream. And we benefit from the positive effect of negative ions whenever we take a shower or walk by the ocean.

When I don't have the time to seek out nature's venues, I create my private wet zone by filling a tub with scented bath salts. A salt soak at the end of the day is a wonderful way to restore oneself and prepare the body for a good night's sleep. Dead Sea salts, rich in restorative minerals, are the most powerful and worth the extra cost. See the Health Resource section for some recommendations. If you're ever short on time and feel depleted, try taking a quick shower using Salt Suds by Origins for the time-management version of a salt soak. This formula contains sea salts and essential oils to relax and purify your body.

3. Earth Power

A Native American woman once explained to me that the Earth is our mother and our friend because it has restorative powers of transmutation. Those who can consciously engage these powers are called shamans. One of their prescriptions for encouraging a blissful-wise-healing state is earth-walking. What's the difference between normal walking and earth-walking? Earth-walking is walking barefoot, mindful of where we step as we seek out the Earth's energies to rebalance us, consciously releasing negative energies and anxieties.

To engage in this practice, visualize drain-like openings on the bottoms of your feet, then imagine pulling out the stopper and allowing your negative emotions—anger, jealousy, anxiety, hostility, turmoil—to pour out of your body, through the feet, and into the ground. Sometimes, I use the analogy of a camera lens that adjusts according to the available light. Think of the imaginary openings on your soles as apertures, replacing negative energy with the healing power of the Earth.

A beach or a grassy meadow is an ideal place to earth-walk, but any field or trail will do. And as my Native American friend likes to say, "Smoother surfaces are easier on tender feet."

If you can't or don't wish to experience Earth's energy through your feet, you can take it in through your senses. Breathe in the fresh air, listen to the sounds of nature, and notice the wind or the calm in the air. Attune your senses to the outdoors where Mother Nature is doing her thing—and will help us do ours if we allow it.

4. Fire Power

Have you ever noticed how relaxed you feel after sitting in a sauna or lazing around a roaring fire? Fire is a powerful tool for clearing and freeing the mind; the whole premise of ashtanga yoga is to stoke the inner fire. A bonfire on the beach is especially healing because you have the essence of water and fire combined. But if a day (or night) at the shore is a dream out of reach, you can still experience the healing powers of fire from the sun. Just a half-hour or so of sunbathing can soothe and heal body and mind. And don't let a little sweat bother you; it's an effective way to rid yourself of toxins and tension. Just be sure, particularly if you're fair-skinned, to slather on the sunscreen and avoid the burning rays in the middle of the day. If you don't have a fireplace, another way to access your fire power is to burn candles. The glow of candlelight always brings a sort of "aahhh" quality to enhance relaxation.

5. Essential Oil Power

The power of aromatherapy is another vehicle for renewal. The ancient Egyptians used essential oils to heal and protect them from the desert sun. Today, we are fortunate to have so many fine brands of these near-magical potions. Clary sage clears the mind and lifts the spirits. Lavender calms and soothes. Rose is relaxing and opens the heart. Rosemary stimulates circulation and energizes. Eucalyptus helps us breathe. Bergamot minimizes depression and helps combat PMS. Lemon is cleansing and clearing. Blue tansy is paradise in a formula blended with other oils. In the United States, doTerra has a vast line of essential oils, (see the Health Resource section) and Young Living has offered aromatherapy products since the '90's. England has high-grade suppliers because they have used essential oils in medical clinics for decades. Single oils are potent and powerful, but blended oils are like perfume with performance. They produce a richer, more complex smell and magnify the impact.

If the idea of wearing oils isn't appealing, you can diffuse essential oils into the air and breathe in the fragrance. A candle made with essential oils is also helpful if it is lit nearby. If oils in any form don't work for you, room fragrance can deliver aromas to help you feel balanced and restored. Bath gels and soaps can also deliver fragrance to sooth you. Moulton Brown has several body wash blends, from Rose Absolute to Eucalyptus, that awaken the senses. (www.moultonbrown.com.)

6. Inner Circle Power

Nothing beats the power of friendship. It's essential to our well-being to have like-minded friends who will support us and help us grow, and whom we can help in turn. Twelve-step programs are a wonderful place to take your emotional baggage if an addiction pattern is present or if family alcoholism is an issue. Al-Anon is the family program associated with Alcoholics Anonymous, and I've never seen such troopers. These people will stand by you and get you back on track no matter how tough your situation.

Churches, synagogues, and temples are also fortresses of spiritual development and companionship. I've been to some that offer such extensive classes that they're almost like a junior college and spiritual center all rolled into one. You'll know you're in the right place when you find yourself among kindred spirits. Another great format for those in the creative arts (or those who aspire to be) are support groups like those that work through *The Artist's Way: A Spiritual Path to Higher Creativity* by Julia Cameron. Cameron's work is tailored to clear out the chaos so you can expand your horizons and creativity. She is the writer who brought Artist's Dates to my life in her groundbreaking bestseller. Even HMOs and hospices offer support groups for those facing illness or loss, which is when we most need inner-circle power. Whenever you find yourself struggling with chaos and internal or external difficulties, this is the time to turn to others. You'll find a sense of calm in togetherness.

7. Family Power

Nothing compares to time with family. There is a history that magically binds us together when we allow the good times to prevail. If you think you come from a dysfunctional-beyond-belief family, cultivate one person in your clan whom you can talk to when you need more than a friend. Just having the same parents or grandparents gives us a commonality we can't share with the outside world. Family members will usually be aware of both our strengths and weaknesses, and the fact they stick by and love us in spite of it all is restorative and reassuring.

I have a favorite aunt from childhood who now lives in Kentucky. Our common link is yoga and our unique approach to life. When we talk about family, so much gets healed. We share a common perspective. We can laugh until we cry and cry until we laugh. In one hour, we can rehash the decades, for we enjoy a special, richly-textured friendship.

8. Breath Power

Here is the one thing in your life you can always control—your breathing. The rate, the depth, the sound, and the location are all within your control. Through yoga, I have learned to take deep, yogic breaths. They have a therapeutic effect because you constrict the opening in your throat, extending the breath by lengthening the time spent breathing in and out. This throat constriction creates a sort of Darth-Vader-like sound that further helps focus your mind on just one thing: the breath you are taking in that moment. Deep, diaphragmatic breaths slow down the brain, oxygenate the body, and create total relaxation.

If I'm highly stressed, I've learned to coax myself into a state of sleep-inducing relaxation with these deep-breathing techniques. When I focus on lengthening each breath, the narrowing-throat sound eases my worries away. Thank you, God, for this built-in, stress-reducing tool; it's so much better than turning to one of our not-so-healthy habits. (Parents of young children whose sleep is often interrupted will find this tool especially helpful.) Here's a quick breathing exercise you can do anywhere. It helps to close your eyes (unless you're behind the wheel), and then visualize your breath as a radiant light filling your body. See the light/breath entering your mouth and spilling down your throat. As the light uses the spine to direct its way through the central core of the body, feel yourself let go and experience a sense of renewal. The more breaths you take, the lighter you feel, and the more energized you become. Continue until you feel filled with light from within. Then enjoy this light moment. As you open your eyes, look into a mirror. See if you don't shine a little brighter!

9. Immune Power

When we get depleted, our immune system joins us. In today's world, with so many viruses and super bugs, you want to be attentive to your immune system as part of the restoration process. The best approach to health is prevention. Giving your immune system support when you are healthy, not sick, is the key that works for me. I've been taking supplements for decades and my favorite immune supplements are RuVital Supplements. (See the Health Resource section.) I also adore Collodial Silver and one another company Bio Nativus has a beautiful kit to keep you healthy during cold and flu season. It includes nose spray, throat spray, ear drops, and hand sanitizer. I use their products to since I travel extensively and enjoy the combination of Silver and Aloe Vera.

10. Clearing Power

Sometimes "clearing" can occur immediately after an earth-walk or a relaxing salt soak, but other times it's not so easy. When we carry resentments and allow anger to rule us, we become heavy from the chaos in our minds and bodies. Clearing ourselves is a way of achieving a calmer state. I often ask people during workshops, "Where do you live?" They usually reply with a geographic location. After I hear several answers, I say, "No, you all live in one place—within your skin."

How clean is that house, the house within?

As someone who works with energy, I find it will sometimes take days to clear myself from the stress of a heavy patient workload. I then have to remind myself that I am clearing my "house" of negative energy, so I keep breathing, walking, oiling, soaking, sunning, and connecting with my inner circle of friends and family until I'm ready to roar again.

We impede our progress when we overexert our bodies and get burned out to achieve some mighty ambition. No glory is worth it if we destroy our health in the process.

I've worked with talented doctors for over a decade. I won't forget the day Doctor Smith told me, "People with unresolved anger and hurts don't heal as quickly, if at all." This was her observation working bedside with cancer patients over decades.

Many cancers might be prevented if people would take time out to share their burdens in the sanctuary of a support group instead of making poor lifestyle choices that send them into the ER. Ignoring aches and pains or masking them with medications can allow cancer to get a foothold at the cellular level. A friend of mine, a wonderful motivational speaker, developed a cancer of the blood that was difficult to detect. He was an expert on time management and gave seminars around the country. But he forgot to keep his life in balance and raced his engines on high for too long. I love this guy and felt so sad that at 57, he hadn't learned how to slow down and nurture himself.

Another example is a client who was an overcommitted father and husband who worked himself into a state of poor health. He needed a kidney transplant at the age of 42 but refused to follow his doctors' instructions during the healing process. Within a year, he was on crutches and in need of one, if not two, hip replacements. He wasn't able to benefit fully from modern medicine because he failed to do his part in restoring his health. Are your accomplishments worth losing your health?

According to Taoist philosophy, our every movement results from the force that directs and orchestrates life. The master is one who yields to this force and allows events to occur, knowing that the master's task is to stay composed and clear. In this clear state of mind and body, we can react with purpose and pleasure, no matter what the circumstance.

I'll never forget the inspiring stories after the tragedy of 9/11 about people who possessed a clear sense of purpose and confidence, even in the midst of grave danger. This is how the Taoist master lives. In the aftermath of a tragedy, we have to take each day and allow the forces to play out without engaging all our projections of fear and doubt. We all have deep, emotional patterns and fears that we must face. Let this book be a wake-up call, offering ways to live at a higher level if we want to achieve purpose and pleasure during times of danger and uncertainty. Whoever said life was a sure thing? But as long as you are alive, your inner house is certain, for it is where you live.

As we move on from creating renewal and restoration, it's time to look at the relationships in your life. What friends and family are helping you create the life you desire and deserve? What relationships are dragging you down? We're starting with your most critical relationship in the world—your relationship with yourself. To love others and receive love, you must first love yourself unconditionally.

Chapter 12

Trusting the Process in Your Life and Relationships

*Tolerance and celebration of individual differences
is the fire that fuels lasting love.*
~Tom Hannah

What is your philosophy on relationships? Do you believe some people come into your life for a reason, a season, or a lifetime? What is your philosophy on trusting the process? By that I mean managing both the rise and fall inherent in all relationships. Relationships—whether with yourself, a demanding boss, a loving partner, or judgmental Aunt Edith—can feel like nirvana or be too toxic to take.

In my experiences in life and through working with my clients, I've come to see that there are no "bad" people, just friends and teachers. Every connection can be a lesson, no matter how painful. You have to put in the time and personal work to unravel the negative aspects and see the blessings hidden within *all* of your relationships. I've lived this philosophy for several decades and have marveled at the tenacity of some relationships and the sheer joy of others.

This chapter focuses on the circular nature of relationships as they ebb and flow, teaching us valuable lessons. In relationships, there can be periods of rapid growth and connectedness followed by fallouts and detachment. I've observed this in my own life and working with others.

Why? When we connect with someone, we are joining our lives with theirs, if only for a moment. Two lives have more opportunities for friction and fallout. Now imagine the ripples that flow through families and offices where groups of people are constantly bumping into one another—pleasantly sometimes, not so nicely other times. It's no wonder those environments are where we often feel the most crisis and conflict.

There is also the complexity of how different people react to turbulent times. Some of us see an opportunity for personal development while others want to stick their heads in the sand. Some people seem programmed for success and more success. Others feel like they never catch a break. Some people can grow and achieve, and that's the note they play best. Others are managing chaos and fallout all the time but are adept at reinventing themselves or others. Some don't risk but also don't stir the pot, so they can be calming. All these different reactions make relationships tricky to maneuver around.

The best mentor in relationships I've known and worked with is Taylor Hartman, author of *The People Code: It's All About Your Innate Motive*. His simple system helps people take an introspective look at their core motive in life and how that influences their relationship styles with others. I still use his personality profiles and endorse his books today. They're useful because relationships are complex, so the solutions need to be simple. If you are looking to do even more relationship work beyond this chapter, I suggest taking a look at his works.

Let's review some tools and techniques to help you navigate choppy relationship waters. The goal is learning balance so you can skillfully maneuver in times of success and stress. I believe resiliency in tough times comes from managing relationship high points with the fallout or obstacles that life throws our way. Let's start with the most important relationship of all: the one with yourself.

Fall in Love with Yourself—First

The first relationship we all have to master is the one we have with ourselves. Only then do we have the compassion and resiliency to join with another soul. I believe we call people into our life. If we're at war with ourselves (overeating, drinking, hiding, lying), we are going to pull people that can either help us out of the dark or drag us deeper. The goal is to master the ebb and flow of your inner world before adding another relationship to the mix.

Eventually, most relationships have to manage the "who is in power" with the "who is right this time" aspect of a partnership. Of course, some relationships don't go down this road, but it's a familiar one to many of us. Most long-term marriages will face this crossroad. And it's especially true if you've experienced early childhood trauma.

All the challenges of childhood become magnified in a partnership. That's why it's so important to take time for an inward reflection and glance in the mirror. It's easy to bring old messages into new relationships, especially if you were negatively labeled as difficult, stupid, spoiled, or worthless as a child. If people said to you: why do you have to be so perfect? Always right? The victim? The bully? The mean girl? These might be patterns and roles that served a purpose in surviving a traumatic childhood but are no longer useful. Even if you came from a healthy family, our roles of the "good one," the "smart one," the "quiet one," and "the baby" could unintentionally seep into our partnerships, where they get amplified.

As I mentioned in Chapter 5: Keys to Calm, most of my family rejected me, except my father. This early childhood trauma set me up to be overly concerned about what other people said or thought about me. The black-sheep role in a family is the one beset with gossip and attack.

The family throws their baggage on that person, so they don't look at their own. This is especially true in an alcoholic or food-obsessed family, where they gossip about those not in the room as they sip or munch their cares away.

Searching for a Destiny

So how did I eventually find love for myself and then another? I decided to get off the street corner of *I Don't Trust You* and *Lonely Street* and take another road to find my future.

When I confessed to my trusted friend Roberta that I was looking for someone, she didn't hesitate a minute to ask, "Are you praying about this?" The thought had never occurred to me! So, I delved in immediately and wrote a prayer treatment. (For how to do this, see Chapter 10: Spiritual Healing Solutions and Prayer Power). My favorite line from the prayer I wrote claimed this:

> *The magnet in my heart is now drawing*
> *my True Love Relationship to me.*

And so, I prayed. I prayed for nine months that I would find my romantic match and soul mate. While I prayed, I worked on my inner world. I sought spiritual healing. I focused on healthy eating and exercise. I meditated and read books, trying to heal what had happened to me as a child. It wasn't always easy, but I kept on praying. In my professional life, men surrounded me. In the food industry, I worked almost exclusively with men, from calling on executive chefs to working with other food brokers, with lots of salesmen sprinkled in too. Not a one asked me out.

But at my favorite grocery store, I kept noticing this one guy who seemed to be everywhere I shopped. Eventually, we struck up a conversation longer than, "Can you tell me where the kale is?" I learned he was a world traveler and worked to live rather than lived to work. One day, he was working the checkout line and put a rosebud in my hand with my receipt. Did I mention roses are my favorites? The next thing I knew, he put his name and phone number on the receipt too!

Of course, I called, and we've been making a life together for the past twenty-five years. We were inseparable after our first date. I married him eighteen months after the first rose! All of the miracles in my life—my husband being one of my biggest—came from raising my awareness with spiritual solutions. That's why this book is filled with so many of these tools and practices.

The biggest lesson I've had in creating lasting, successful relationships is that I had to *get myself* before I could *get another*. Once you live to express yourself fully in this life, you will have to master relationships. If you are ready to find love or start anew and begin again, here are the five steps to take:

1) Open Your Heart to Love

I know how simple this sounds, but it's not. When you open your heart to love, you give it out in generous servings to strangers, neighbors, mail carriers, and the public. You offer a smile easily and give compliments. It's small steps that break down the barriers you've built around your heart. Learning to flirt is a big deal for some who have been heartbroken.

2) Be Curious About Anyone that Gives Attention to YOU

This doesn't mean that you date everyone who smiles at you on the street. But start to notice when you find a man who makes you laugh or an exciting woman who makes you smile. Be curious what brings people to you and how you attract (or don't attract) attention. Look for motives. "Oh, this person is going out of the way to be kind, but why?" Start to notice if you can tell who is single and putting out a vibe that appeals to you. Are they seeking friendship or business advice? We have to learn our motives in life, but it's a healthy study to see if you can look into others' motives too. One of my dear friends, a retired nurse of forty years, Sandra, says all the time, "We all get used in life; after all, we are here to serve."

3) Don't Fall Head Over Heels

If you are lonely and looking for romance, friendship, or business partners, don't go overboard, or you could drown. People don't need to know everything about you all at once. Good things take time, so pace yourself. Friends and lovers should have a mutual exchange of interest and energy. The same is true with business associates and partnerships: mutual respect is key. If that is lacking, then the relationship won't be as lasting or fulfilling.

4) Trust the Attraction and Orchestration

Falling in love is like a weaving process. It's a personal tapestry where each interaction becomes a thread. Staying in the moment is great if something special arrives. So, let the threads mingle. Know that when the threads are ready, the picture will come together as words, feelings, and gestures. Trust that your chemistry will become joyously clear. This pertains to friendships as well as romance. Surround yourself with people who bring out your magic, not your madness.

5) Prioritize Partnership and Success Will Follow

All grow-getters eventually learn that true growth comes from collaboration. We can't do this life thing alone, not in our personal lives or in the business world. Recently, a business associate called with birthday wishes. The first thing she said was, "I don't have time to talk." Suddenly, I felt put off by this call. One word could have changed the flavor of the conversation. If she'd only said, "I don't have *long* to talk." Maybe this sounds too sensitive, but you'd be surprised how abrupt energy doesn't register as caring energy. If you call people and say that you don't have time to talk, you aren't prioritizing them. You're just checking in. So, carve out time to let people know, in business or personal relationships, that they matter. The new ways of communication (especially with social media) have made more areas where we can build bridges to be connected, rather than rafts that drift apart.

Look for Those Relationships That Feel Like a Safety Net

When people come from dysfunctional family systems or experience Adverse Childhood Events (ACEs), it's going to show up later in life when they attempt to get into a relationship, or if they never get involved in a relationship, period. Having experienced abuse, rejection, or betrayal early in life, those souls are naturally going to be wary of getting close to or trusting others. If this is you or someone you love, don't feel alone with this pain. There are plenty of people to meet if you find loneliness your constant companion. When you decide you don't want to live this way, then start to change! That means taking chances and finding the best way to engage.

As if this life isn't complex enough, we have to ideally strive to achieve finding *safety-net relationships* in both our professional and personal lives. Many people with successful home lives can't seem to climb the corporate business ladder because the shark tank is too threatening. Conversely, many with high levels of professional status can swim with the sharks and find it a wonderful challenge, but don't have a stable home life or significant other. Wherever you are in this paradigm, the goal is to get to a place where you feel: *I have all I need.* Expectations for success are met, and disappointments are managed. When you get here, it feels safe. That's contentment.

Trusting the Good in Grief to Find Relief

Within our lives we experience many losses, from job transitions to relationship "surprises." After each loss and setback, we have to reconfigure ourselves to adjust. How do you go from disappointed and distressed to rekindling your spirit and reappointing yourself for a greater good?

In my role as a patient advocate, I would often be comforting loved ones right as their spouses passed away. No one had to tell me to bring my A-game on those darkest days. I knew this was a defining moment for the loved ones. The blessing was in finding that these pinnacle moments were mutual. I remember all my patients on these occasions because the vulnerability of the human spirit was so exposed.

Once, I was working with a retired New York City police officer whose wife had died very suddenly from complications with liver cancer. She was walking around the hospital chatting with others at lunch, missed dinner because of no appetite, and was in Heaven by midnight. It was fast; most of the medical professionals didn't see her demise coming. Which means all of us were in shock, trying to help the family after the passing.

I knew my job was to help this tough guy shift his grief to the gift of time: the time he'd had at the end with his wife, not to mention their twenty-plus years of marriage. My intention was to assist him from grief-stricken toward finding some golden strand to help him get through the day. This is where the trust comes in. We must all trust that there are golden strands to find, if only we look. This is what we are all asked to do in chaotic times.

When I approached him, his resistance was palpable, "I don't know if I want to sit down with you because I might feel things I don't want to feel."

"I'm only here to support you. If you want to sit outside, we can talk. If not, you can stay here in the reception area," I said.

I was so honored that he followed me and took those first few steps toward grief and healing. As we talked about the final details of his wife's life, tears filled his eyes. It was like letting some steam out of a kettle, so it doesn't boil over. He needed to begin to feel his grief, even if it was only for five minutes. It was a victory to express even a few tears, so he didn't push all his grief away after suffering such a major loss. I was able to plant the seed as his tears fell, that as with all relationships, his season with his wife might be over, but he had to get the strength to move on.

Grief is part of the process of rising above the chaos. We've been conditioned to believe expressing grief is causing havoc, but that's not the case. Appropriate grief has to be expressed and healed. It's a bridge we cross within ourselves to gain our footing in life. Male or female, young or old, you have to get equipped to handle this mysterious thing called grief. It's a strong emotion that can turn into depression or unhealthy behaviors if we don't allow it to surface.

What Happened to My Glorious Job?

We've talked a lot about personal losses, but professional setbacks pack a punch too. When the status of a job relationship changes, we have to trust the process of discomfort to adjust our sails. These changes are due to any number of variables: a new boss or workmates, new owner-ship, burnout, abuse by management or co-workers, or it's just no longer the right fit. You can be in a fabulous job, and the company gets bought out. The new owners don't see you as the IT professional they need, and the promising future you always had is gone. Work upheavals are often out of our control. What we can control is how we process the loss and the lessons it will teach us.

When it comes to doing your grief work, the longer you've been in the position, the longer you have to honor the loss. You've got to grieve the change in relationship and status in the company. Some people stuff down these major and minor losses, like the New York policeman wanted to, and bottle them up. But that's not trusting the process. The *only* way out is through it. Let the tears, anger, and lower feelings surface; let them be honored, so you can move on. Remember the example of fear storms in Chapter 2: Categories of Chaos? Well, we can have grief storms too.

Savannah, one of my coaching clients, lost her mother and was trying to keep busy during the first Christmas season without her. I could hear her almost hyperventilating as she reviewed all these plans and people she was going to be with. I understood this grief reaction. Expressing your grief doesn't mean crying alone, cloistered away from society. It's a balance that I'm trying to convey between letting the tears flow and then drying your eyes, so you'll laugh harder when something funny occurs. Grief is a roller-coaster ride with many rainbows after the tears have cleared. But when you prevent grief, you also block your joy. Savannah heeded my advice and spent a day alone before the holiday commitments with family and friends to be with her feelings, just as they were.

We All Have Relationship Wounds

Why do we think we have to be tough to survive all the chaos and lessons in life? Maybe it's due to the early survival skills of our ancestors. But we need to cry more than we allow and laugh even more at the absurdities of life. Emotions get blocked if we don't allow ourselves to feel them. It's a common theme in this book: if you suppress your negative emotions, you block the good ones.

I always learn through my clients and my work. So, before I could finish this book, I decided to make a pre-Thanksgiving trip from my home in San Diego to visit my mother at her senior care facility out of state. While it wasn't a warm and fuzzy relationship while I was growing up, now that Mom was 90, I knew there were not a lot of holidays left.

I always do three-day visits when seeing my mother. I wanted to honor that my family gave me life, shelter, education, many talents, and lots of glorious examples of what to do. But when it came to love and nurturing from Mom, not so much.

Mom is now frail, and her memories are sketchy, but she's not by any stretch already gone. During my stay, there were no thank-you's for the gifts I brought, or for the time and money it had taken to visit. I knew not to expect them, but I still noticed their absence. Instead, she took pleasure in criticizing me: for not staying longer and for not doing and being enough. She even made a "fat" comment that would have derailed me in my youth.

But I smiled through it all, knowing that she could no longer hurt me. I had mastered a life lesson because I trusted the process that meant one day I would be healed from my mother or any family members' rejection. The circumstances had not changed; I had. So, I kissed her goodbye on day three and went flying back to San Diego.

Lessons Within Lessons: Pay Attention Please

Leaving my mom and heading to the airport, it seemed the lesson of love and forgiveness wasn't over. In all my years of traveling on airplanes, I never had the screaming-baby flight where you are bombarded with the baby's cries and upset parents. That changed on this trip! I had back-to-back connections to San Diego, and I had a screaming baby directly behind me to start the flight.

I felt the parents' embarrassment and how hard this was on them too, while I heard the child's wailing behind me. Suddenly, the baby threw up everywhere, and now the parents were humiliated. Amidst the chaos behind my seat, it was like an Angel tapped me on my shoulder. The message was: *Your mother may not have adored you with words or loving looks, but she did love you through her deeds and the sacrifice of a mother. Appreciate her!* It was a life-affirming moment that put the whole trip in perspective.

The last connection of the trip was ahead of me and I assumed I had received my Angel lesson for the day. I boarded the next flight and this time found myself seated next to a three-month-old baby. The infant was sitting almost on my shoulder because of the way the mother was holding her on my side of her seat. Of course, it had to be a baby girl, right?

So, I started talking to the mother. "How old is your baby?" Then I inquired, "So what's it like being a mother? Do you enjoy it?"

"It's so amazing!" said this beautiful mother who was in her late 30's. She kept gazing at her daughter and said, "I love her so much." I watched the two of them lovingly looking at each other for hours. I was so happy to be in the presence of all this mother-daughter love.

Then my higher self/Angel tapped me on my shoulder again. *Yes, this relationship with your mother was a difficult situation in your life. Be at peace now.* It felt like I received permission to tell this story here. I realized even as a baby, my mother didn't have the glow of love like I was witnessing. Mom and I just didn't have this relationship. But guess what? My life was and is amazing, and I love her anyway!

Whatever the Question, Acceptance Is the Answer

Hopefully, with whatever you've got to resolve in your life today, you can find a way to trust the process and not feel like a victim to other people or circumstances. Dr. Paul Ohliger, a writer and helper to humanity, wrote his version of Acceptance as quoted in the Alcoholics Anonymous "Big Book":

> Acceptance is the answer to all my problems today. When I am disturbed, it is because I find some person, place, thing, or situation—some fact of my life—unacceptable to me, and can find no serenity until I accept that person, place, thing or situation as being exactly the way it is supposed to be at this moment.

This reminds me, relationships are like the yin and yang symbol with the black and white halves and a spot of the opposite color contained within. When we get profoundly rejected, no one wants to have that kind of resentment or darkness to rule their life. But like the yin and yang symbol, I know that there is light in the darkness because I've field-tested this truth. Even the most saintly, perfect lives have a bit of darkness in their light. It's called the human condition.

Remember when you can't get things right with another, your first job is to resolve your internal chaos and accept the situation as being the Universe's lesson for you and your growth. Don't just travel down any path to engage with a problem. Stop fighting it and find a way of getting out of feeling overwhelmed.

Here is a simple three-step process I often use.

First, I want to address my situation squarely. That is my acceptance. I have to acknowledge an external problem that has shown up and get ready to find a new perspective or solution.

Second, I'm going to put all my might into healing or resolving this belief, wound, upset, habit, or threat to my security until it's resolved. This takes action.

Third, I've got to trust chaos, the great teacher who always delivers me to greater possibilities when I stop the blame game and move up in my approach to life. I have to thank the problem for showing up and honor myself for wanting to rise above it. This gives me freedom.

This is the path I take, and I recommend others follow, for health and sanity: Trust the process and put all your energy into the solution, not the problem. This new way of living can yield fantastic results. I've seen it with my patients and clients and been blessed to experience this peaceful healing from chaos many times over. If someone is rude to you or unjustly attacks you, you don't have to fight back. Revenge is a lower expression of living and causes chaos. Living right, and loving yourself and others no matter what, is the definition of Rising Above the Chaos. When your internal chaos is in check, you can master whatever the world is delivering to you today. The reward for right living is simple; it's living right!

Let's Stay Connected!

'm so honored we have been on this journey together. It is with joy and love that I share much of my life's work with you. There is no right or wrong answer in how to use this book. I hope you sample a little of everything. If something resonated and sparked an interest or feeling, I hope you dive deeper.

In my world, these have been the building blocks that enriched my soul and created a connection within and outside of myself to something of significance. Let them be the foundation upon which you create your most meaningful, connected, and grow-getter life.

I hope the next time chaos, our greatest teacher, knocks on the door, you'll invite him or her in, now knowing the gifts they bear. This mind shift is the most potent message of the book. I don't wish you troubled times, but remember that when they come, I'm here to help guide you through the dark valley to the summit where you will stand in your new light and glory.

Please know that the tools in this book are now yours to keep. I hope you reap the rewards for the rest of your life as you first transform yourself and then the world!

You can have a playful attitude in searching for the solutions that work for you. Just know that the rest are at the ready when you need them. Different times of disruption in life may call for new solutions. What worked with one crisis might not be the best fit for the next. That's where your newly acquired self-knowledge pays off.

Please be patient with yourself and your progress. Perfection is not required. By taking even a few small steps toward self-reflection and insight, you are developing your rise-above-the-chaos muscles.

On those days when self-care is needed, but the boss or kids are calling you away, think of me cheering you on to take that much-needed walk on the beach, bite of an organic apple, or acupuncturist appointment. I hope you honor yourself as much as I do.

I've so loved thinking about you as I wrote this book, dear reader. I've prayed for your healing, and that this book would find its way into your hands when you needed it most. It's been a roller-coaster ride, but I wouldn't trade it for the world. I've held you close to my heart and will miss you. As I close this book, it's a bittersweet goodbye.

But I'm also excited because I know you will use your newfound calm and gifts of self-knowledge to transform your world. You can become a catalyst for change in your family, workplace, and community. We've never needed you more, and I can't wait to watch the ripples grow.

Yours in health, gratitude, and love,

Carolyn Gross

I want to invite you to continue this journey with me by visiting www.carolyngross.com or www.creativelifesolutions.com website. For specific solutions mentioned in this book visit www.riseabovethechaos.com. These sites will detail my calendar of events, coaching programs, blog, and health products. I've also designed an annual Rise above the Chaos retreat, so email us at info@creativelifesolutions.com if you are interested in learning more. It would be an honor to meet in person, and the sites will list conferences and book signings across the country.

Here are my social media links, if that's how you'd prefer to stay in touch.

Facebook: facebook.me/cg.riseabovethechaos

Twitter: twitter.com/carolyngrosscls

LinkedIn: linkedin.com/in/carolyngross/

About the Author

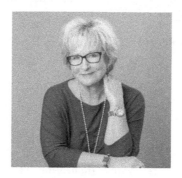

For over twenty-five years Carolyn Gross has been serving others with her expertise in self-care and health care. She plays several roles in the helping professions, including: professional speaker, patient and health advocate, and author of four wellness books as featured on *ABC*, *NBC*, and *Lifetime TV*.

When she wrote her first book, *Staying Calm in the Midst of Chaos*, before the events of September 11th, she began an eighteen-month tour for the book. The tour ended when she found a lump in her breast and was diagnosed with Stage Three Breast Cancer.

In 2003, against the odds, she stared down a diagnosis of infiltrating ductal carcinoma, and chose to keep her breast using Immunotherapy, Chemo, and Radiation. As a trained professional speaker and past president of the National Speakers Association in San Diego, her career took a dramatic turn when she went from stage-side to bed-side. She became a patient advocate and spokesperson for Immunotherapy and then wrote her next two books on Cancer Recovery and Immunotherapy: *Treatable and Beatable: Healing Cancer without Surgery* and her co-authored book, *Breaking the Cancer Code.*

Working with cancer patients and their families for over a decade proved to be a grindstone to sharpen her skills and find solutions to help people rise above the chaos. This latest book is her return to the work she loves, as a motivational speaker, spa and wellness retreat facilitator, and people developer, i.e. life coach.

Dedicated to her craft, she is a twenty-year member of the National Speakers Association, and a popular keynote speaker at conventions and health related events across the United States and Canada. Carolyn has facilitated spa retreats and women's wellness programs for some of the most exclusive spas in the world including: The Golden Door, Hilton Waikoloa, Rancho La Puerta, Cal-A-Vie, and Ojai Valley Inn & Spa.

She dedicates herself to helping people by combining creative life solutions with wellness principles. Her multi-faceted approach to managing the sea of change we live in, has been an inspiration to help people make informed decisions in challenging times.

She enjoys living in the San Diego area with her husband Bryan and golden doddle Nibbles, a.k.a. her boys! She loves teaching, coaching, live performances, music and the arts, nature hikes, mineral springs, yoga, and Whole Foods.

Her motto: "Life can be fulfilling no matter what surprises chaos, the great teacher, sends our way. Just stay focused on positive outcomes, keep your child-like joy (wish upon a star) and take every step possible in the direction of your dreams."

Health Resources

Art of Raising Frequency

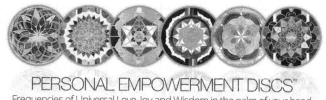

PERSONAL EMPOWERMENT DISCS™
Frequencies of Universal Love, Joy and Wisdom in the palm of your hand

The Personal Empowerment Discs are high vibrational healing tools that interact with us to support the human biofield. The geometric designs and vibrations help us allow positive frequencies of love, joy, and harmony to blossom while diminishing negative vibrations of fear, anger and hopelessness. For health professionals and practitioners, the Chakra Healing Discs are amazing. Both sets are highly beneficial for creating healing in the human biofield. Anyone can benefit from adding these unique discs and artwork to their treatment protocols and offices, stimulating transformational energetic shifts that create a sustained movement toward vibrant health. Most professionals believe it takes their healing work and practice to a whole new level. You can get a discount when you call or email our office for a special code. (760) 741-2762 or directly purchase online https://www. crystalwingshealingart.com/ using RAC15

Body Care: Essential Oils doTerra

These blends are nothing short of miraculous. If you'd like to sample the wizardry of doTeRRA, you may call 1-800-411-8151 or email us to get full instructions and recommendations at info@creativelifesolutions. com. Here are the oils I recommend for stress-related conditions.

Name of Oil	Blend	Amt.	Benefits
Balance	Grounding Blend (warm & woody)	15ml.	Balances mind, body and emotions
Deep Blue	Soothing (minty & camphoraceous)	5ml.	Soothing and cooling blend Comforting part of a massage
DigestZen	Digestive Blend (spicy, sweet, minty, licorice)	15ml.	Can be used internally to support healthy digestion Soothes occasional stomach upset, bloating, gas
On Guard	Protective Blend (warm, spicy, camphoraceous, woody)	15ml.	Supports immune system Antioxidant
Elevation	Joyful Blend (floral, sweet, citrus)	15ml.	Elevates mood and increases vitality
Zendocrime	Detoxification Blend (herbaceous, pungent, floral)	15ml.	Supports healthy liver function Purifying and detoxifying to the body's system
Lavender	*Lavandula angustifolia*	15ml.	Soothes skin irritations Can be taken internally to reduces anxious and tension Promote peaceful sleeps

Origins

One of the best "feel good" stores around is Origins. In stores, you are encouraged to sample the various creams, bath gels, and salt scrubs. Just visiting a store is relaxing in itself. Recommended products are Peace of Mind on the Spot gel, Ginger Body Scrub and Salt Rub, Clean Comfort and Salt Subs bath gels, Ginger Soufflé body cream, and Ginger Burst body wash. To purchase call Origins at 1-800-ORIGINS (1-800-674-4467) or visit their website at www.origins.com.

Massage and Alternative Health Helpful Websites

Alexander Technique

The Alexander Technique International's website (www.ati-net.com) will help you locate a trained instructor. For further questions, you can email them through their website, or mail to PO Box 3948, Parker, CO 80134, or give them a call at (303) 482-2092.

CranioSacral therapy

For more information on obtaining a CranioSacral Therapist call International Alliance of Health Educators at 1-800-311-9204 or visit their website www.iahe.com for a variety of healing modalities.

Lymph Drainage Therapy

To locate a Lymph Drainage Therapist or purchase Dr. Bruno Chikly's book, *Silence Waves: Theory and Practice of Lymph Drainage Therapy*, contact International Alliance of Healthcare Educators (IAHE) at 1-800-311-9204. You can also find the book on www.Amazon.com.

Minerals and Supplements

4 reasons why minerals are important to maintain your health:

1. Earth soils are Mineral Deficient, and they help with Vitamin Utilization
2. Body Functions are improved by Electrolytes
3. Proper Hydration and Nutrition Minimizes Anxiety and Depression
4. Prevent Premature Aging especially in the bones, skin, nails, teeth, muscles, nerves, ligaments, and tendons.

Bio Nativus

Bio Nativus is committed to harvesting rich and beneficial minerals and supplements. They consult with many medical professionals and constantly test their products in numerous clinical labs. I would recommend the *Silvera 24 ppm Solution Kit* for cold and flu season. I like the formulas of the products in this kit, because of their main ingredients are one hundred percent Purified Silver and liquid Aloe Vera.

You can place your order on their website bionativus.com or call them at 1-888-628-4887.

Ruvital Supplements

Ruvital has been developed after thirty years of research and clinical application. The ingredients of their products are of the highest nutritional quality and are produced with customers' health in mind. Their formulas are aimed at preventing disease and strengthening health. For those with serious chronic conditions, these are amazing to know about.

Here is the list of supplements:

Supplement Name	Benefits
BR: Connection (Brain Enhancer)	Improves Brain Functioning, Mind Concentration and Memory Development Reduce Depression Inhibits mental retardation

CellPro (Stem Cell Enhancer)	Reinforces and Supports the Immune System Restores and Strengthens Organs and Tissue Beneficial for Memory Function with Neuro-Regenerators Promotes the release of stem cells
Immucan	Supports Immune System and Memory Regulates Blood Pressure Fights Allergies
Immune Enhance	Strengthens the Immune System Supports Digestive Tract Function Strong Anti-oxidant
Progland for Men or Women	Helps repair Cells and get Energy Promotes good Glandular Production, Memory and Metabolic Functioning

You can place the order through our office Creative Life Solutions www.creativelifesolutions.com contact order form or by visiting their website at http://www.ruvitalsupplements.com. If you have questions email info.cls@aol.com give us a call (760) 741-2762.

Sea Salt

Using mineral and dead sea salts is a wonderful remedy for people with insomnia. A salt soak before bed leads to restful sleep because it purifies and relaxes. BathTherapy and Masada Dead Sea Salts are available at most health food stores. For high-powered bathers, I recommend Kerstin Florin Mineral Kur bath salts. If you are getting a cold, these salts boost the immune system. For information on where to purchase these mineral salts and creams call 888-537-7846.

For a therapeutic bath salt that fills the skin with its powerful ingredients and a restorative spa experience from home, I recommend Ahava Eucalyptus Dead Sea Mineral Bath. It helps with hydrating and detoxifying the skin. You can order it from their website at www.ahava.com.

Another product of bath soak that will leave you satisfied all night after the bath is Elemis Aching Musle Super Soak. This bath soak is rich in minerals. The ingredients relieve body stress and purify the skin with aromatherapy powers of lavender, rosemary, and chamomile. To purchase this product, you can go to their website at www.elemis.com.

Tea

Therapeutic benefits of drinking tea: It's an antioxidant, contains less caffeine than coffee, and is helpful to stimulate the immune system and metabolism.

Art of Tea

Art of Tea offers top tier organic tea (USDA Organic) and selects botanicals. Directly sourcing their teas and botanicals means their teas are innovative and premium quality to ensure a memorable Art of Tea experience. All of their teas are crafted using the 5000-year-old tradition from signature organic loose leaf teas, organic iced teas, and tea sachets. Their intention is to make the experience of drinking artisan tea more fun and interactive.

I recommend their Wellness Teas section if you need teas for balancing and calming. They offer different flavors and health benefits that you can choose from.

To place the order, you can check out their website at https://www.artoftea.com or by phone: 1-877-268-8327.

Health Websites for further exploration:
Adverse Childhood Experiences:
www.childwelfare.gov
www.samhsa.gov

For nutrition and health facts:
    health.gov/
    www.nia.nih.gov/health
    familydoctor.org

References

Chapter 1

"Stress Effects on the Body." American Psychological Association. Accessed February 01, 2019. https://www.apa.org/helpcenter/stress/effects-nervous.aspx.

Chapter 3

Burgess, Lana. "Left Brain vs. Right Brain: Characteristics, Functions, and Myths." Medical News Today. Accessed February 01, 2019. https://www.medicalnewstoday.com/articles/321037.php.

Coles, Paul, Tony Cox, Chris Mackey, and Simon Richardson, eds. "The Toxic Terabyte." *IBM Global Technology Services*, July 2016. Accessed January 26, 2018. doi:10.18411/d-2016-154.

Rodgerson, Thomas E. *Spirituality, Stress & You*. New York: Paulist Press, 1994.

Schilling, David Russell. "Knowledge Doubling Every 12 Months, Soon to Be Every 12 Hours." Industry Tap. June 13, 2017. Accessed February 01, 2019. http://www.industrytap.com/knowledge-doubling-every-12-months-soon-to-be-every-12-hours/3950.

Chapter 5

"Adverse Childhood Experiences." Substance Abuse and Mental Health
    Services Administration| SAMHSA. July 09, 2018. Accessed
    February 01, 2019. https://www.samhsa.gov/capt/practicing-
    effective-prevention/prevention-behavioral-health/adverse-
    childhood-experiences.

Bethell, Christina D et al. "Methods to Assess Adverse Childhood Expe-
    riences of Children and Families: Toward Approaches to Promote
    Child Well-being in Policy and Practice" *Academic pediatrics* vol.
    17,7S (2017): S51-S69.

Chapter 6

Hobbs, Charles R. *Time Power*. New York: Harper & Brothers, 1988.

Chapter 7

"The Original Renewable Energy Source." Federal Occupational
    Health. Accessed February 01, 2019. https://foh.psc.gov/calendar/
    nutrition.html.

Gross, Carolyn, and Geronimo Rubio, MD. *Breaking The Cancer Code: A
    Revolutionary Approach To Reversing Cancer.* Xlibris Corporation, 2013.

Sheppard, Kay. *Food Addiction: The Body Knows*. Deerfield Beach, FL:
    Health Communications, 1993.

Weil, Andrew, MD. "Does Milk Cause Cancer? - Ask Dr. Weil."
    DrWeil.com. February 03, 2017. Accessed February 01, 2019.
    https://www.drweil.com/health-wellness/body-mind-spirit/cancer/
    does-milk-cause-cancer/.

Chapter 8

"Walk Your Way to Fitness." Mayo Clinic. December 14, 2018.
    Accessed February 01, 2019. https://www.mayoclinic.org/
    healthy-lifestyle/fitness/in-depth/walking/art-20046261.

Berkeley Wellness. "Mind-Body Exercise: Tai Chi and Yoga." University of California Berkeley Wellness. March 23, 2016. Accessed February 01, 2019. http://www.berkeleywellness.com/healthy-mind/mind-body/article/mind-body-exercise-tai-chi-and-yoga.

Department of Health & Human Services. "Swimming - Health Benefits." Better Health Channel. August 30, 2013. Accessed February 01, 2019. https://www.betterhealth.vic.gov.au/health/healthyliving/swimming-health-benefits.

Fioranelli, Enrico. "5 Types of Strength Training: Which Is Right for You?" YogiApproved™. August 17, 2015. Accessed February 01, 2019. https://www.yogiapproved.com/health-wellness/5-types-of-strength-training/.

Gottfried, Sara, MD. *Younger A Breakthrough Program to Reset Your Genes, Reverse Aging, and Turn Back the Clock 10 Years*. New York Times, 2017.

Gupta, Sanjay, MD. "The Best Anti-Aging Medicine? Exercise." Stroke Center - EverydayHealth.com. June 17, 2015. Accessed February 01, 2019. https://www.everydayhealth.com/news/best-anti-aging-medicine-exercise.

Harvard Health Publishing. "The Top 5 Benefits of Cycling." Harvard Health Blog. August 2016. Accessed February 01, 2019. https://www.health.harvard.edu/staying-healthy/the-top-5-benefits-of-cycling.

Loria, Kevin. "8 Key Ways Running Can Transform Your Body and Brain." Business Insider. May 27, 2018. Accessed February 01, 2019. https://www.businessinsider.com/health-benefits-of-running-2018-4.

Myers, Johnathan. "Exercise and Cardiovascular Health." AHA Journals. January 07, 2003. Accessed February 01, 2019. https://www.ahajournals.org/doi/full/10.1161/01.cir.0000048890.59383.8d.

Warburton, D. E., C. W. Nicol, and S. S. Bredin. "Health Benefits of Physical Activity: The Evidence." Current Neurology and Neurosci-

ence Reports. March 14, 2006. Accessed February 01, 2019. http://
www.ncbi.nlm.nih.gov/pubmed/16534088.

Weingus, Leigh. "Does Exercise Help Reverse the Effects of Aging?"
Mindbodygreen. March 20, 2017. Accessed February 01, 2019.
https://www.mindbodygreen.com/0-29265/does-exercise-help-
reverse-the-effects-of-aging.html.

Chapter 9

Coppola, Gloria. "Lomi Lomi Massage: The Art of Hawaiian Sacred
Healing." Massage Magazine. May 31, 2018. Accessed February
01, 2019. https://www.massagemag.com/lomilomi-hawaiian-
massage-87100/).

Winner, Jay. *Take the Stress out of Your Life: A Medical Doctors Proven
Program to Minimize Stress and Maximize Health*. Cambridge:
Da Capo Press, 2008.

Chapter 11

"Laughter Yoga International - Health, Happiness, World Peace."
Laughter Yoga University. Accessed February 01, 2019. https://
laughteryoga.org/).

Batmanghelidj, F. *Your Body's Many Cries for Water*. Place of Publication
Not Identified: Tagman Press, 2004.